AF707356

HEAL

HEAL

Your Recovery Blueprint with 100+ Healing Recipes for Injury & Surgery

Kami Parsa, MD

Copyright © 2026 Kami Parsa, MD

Heal: Your Recovery Blueprint
with 100+ Healing Recipes
for Injury & Surgery

Edited by Natasha Vera

Art Direction by Morgane Leoni

Cover Image, Photographs & Illustration © Adobe Stock

ISBN 979-8-9932412-2-7 (hardcover)
ISBN 979-8-9932412-0-3 (paperback)

Disclaimer

This book is not intended as a substitute for consultation with a licensed practitioner. The recipes and dietary suggestions offered in this book are intended for informational purposes. Please note that the suggestions and practices outlined in this guide are based on general principles and may not be suitable for every individual. Personalized advice from your own qualified healthcare professional is recommended. The use of this book implies your acceptance of this disclaimer.

I dedicate this book to my incredible wife, Kathryn,
and our wonderful children, Sofi and Aston.
You are my greatest joy, my inspiration,
and my unwavering foundation.
You mean the world to me.

TABLE OF CONTENTS

INTRODUCTION

Welcome to *Heal: Your Recovery Blueprint with 100+ Healing Recipes for Injury & Surgery*. Whether you're preparing for surgery or navigating the recovery process, this guide is here to support you every step of the way. Surgery can be a daunting experience, but one of the most powerful tools at your disposal is something you encounter every day: food.

The relationship between nutrition and healing is profound. The food you eat before and after surgery can significantly influence how quickly and effectively your body recovers. From reducing inflammation to rebuilding tissues, the right diet can help minimize complications, speed up recovery, and improve your overall outcome.

As some of you may know, I am an oculoplastic surgeon, and I've had the privilege of caring for patients for over twenty years here in Beverly Hills, California. As a surgeon, I've performed thousands of surgeries and have witnessed countless patients go through the healing process. Some recover quickly, while others take a bit longer. The human body is a miracle, and although everyone eventually heals, the pace and manner of recovery vary from person to person.

For many years, like most surgeons, I believed that mastering my surgical technique was the key to ensuring the best outcomes for my patients. I spent thousands of hours perfecting my skills, developing, and publishing new minimally-invasive surgical techniques for oculofacial plastic surgery, such as my signature trifecta and quadfecta lift procedures. I was confident that this technical expertise was the most critical factor in patient recovery.

However, it wasn't until I experienced an injury myself that I discovered the profound impact that nutrition and diet have on healing and recovery. A few years ago, while playing catch with my son, I accidentally suffered a mallet injury, tearing the distal ligament on my middle finger. Two of my hand surgeon colleagues recommended surgery, which would involve placing two pins in my finger for three months to stabilize it and allow proper healing. Although this was my non-dominant hand, the surgery meant I would be unable to operate for at least three months—a daunting prospect for someone who lives for the operating room.

Desperate for an alternative, I embarked on an obsessive deep dive into every peer-reviewed academic paper on healing published over the past twenty years. This research led me down a rabbit hole that eventually became the foundation for this book. To make a long story short, I was able to avoid surgery by using two wooden popsicle sticks to stabilize my finger and, more importantly, by completely changing my diet. Remarkably, my injury healed within two months, allowing me to continue working without interruption. The lessons I learned from this experience were priceless, and I immediately began incorporating every aspect of them into my patients' healing journeys.

Little did I know when writing this book that I would soon become my own case study. As I was completing these chapters, life presented me with a profound twist of fate. Through a routine screening, I discovered that I had a genetic heart condition requiring open heart surgery. In what felt like divine timing, the very research I had compiled for this book—intended to help others—suddenly became my personal roadmap for recovery.

In those moments after receiving my diagnosis, I experienced the same anxiety and uncertainty that I've seen in countless patients' eyes over my years of practice. But I also had something many don't: a comprehensive understanding of how nutrition and lifestyle choices could optimize my body's ability to heal.

I followed the principles outlined in this book to the letter—preparing my body nutritionally before surgery, working closely with my medical team, and implementing the recovery strategies I've detailed in these pages. The results were remarkable. Despite undergoing major open heart surgery, I was discharged from the hospital after only four days (while the average is eight days) and am healing exceptionally well six weeks post-operation as I write these words.

This unexpected journey has transformed this book from professional guidance into a deeply personal testimony. Every recommendation, every nutritional strategy, and every recovery tip has been filtered not just through my experience as a surgeon, but now also through my perspective as a patient who has faced a serious health challenge.

In this guide, we'll explore the science behind healing through nutrition. You'll learn about the key nutrients that play a vital role in recovery, how to prepare your body before surgery, and what to eat during those crucial days and weeks after your procedure. Whether you're facing a minor outpatient surgery or a major operation, this guide offers practical, evidence-based advice to help you heal faster and feel better sooner.

We'll also address common challenges, such as managing appetite loss, combating fatigue, and dealing with post-surgery complications like constipation or inflammation—all through the lens of nutrition. You'll learn practical, evidence-based strategies to support your recovery and help your body heal more efficiently.

One of the most exciting parts of this book is the collection of healing recipes. During my research, I discovered and gathered recipes from a variety of sources, including talented chefs who share my passion for nutritious, healing foods. This extensive recipe section proves that healthy eating doesn't have to be boring or bland. From protein-rich breakfasts that support tissue repair to anti-inflammatory dinner options and nutrient-dense desserts, these recipes demonstrate that making good nutritional choices can be delicious and satisfying. Whether you're a culinary enthusiast or someone who simply wants straightforward, healing meals, you'll find options that nourish your body while delighting your taste buds.

Ultimately, this guide is about empowerment. By understanding how food can support your recovery, you take an active role in your healing journey.

Surgery is just one step on the path to recovery—what you do before and after can make all the difference.

As you read this guide, know that these aren't just theoretical concepts—they are practical tools that supported my own healing and recovery during one of the most challenging periods of my life. My sincere hope is that they will do the same for you, whatever surgical journey you may be facing.

Let's embark on this journey together and discover how the right diet can help you heal and thrive.

1

The Miracle of Healing: Evolution, Survival, and the Body's Repair Process

I'm going to tell you a story—but don't worry, I'll keep it as brief as possible. It's a story that began approximately four billion years ago. It's the story of you, me, and all life on this beautiful planet we call Earth. But before we dive into that, I want to take you back to a specific moment in my life when I fell in love with science and found a deeper sense of spirituality. You might be wondering what that has to do with healing. Trust me, it's all connected.

The year was 1995, and I was a freshman at UCLA, sitting in my Intro to Biology class. As some of you might remember, biology can sometimes feel like a string of facts to memorize—long Latin names and processes that don't seem to have much relevance to daily life. But then, the professor said something that changed everything for me: "Did you know we carry within us the genetic code for the wings of the fruit fly, Drosophila? It's part of the inactive code in our DNA called introns. We shared a common ancestor with the fruit fly around 700 million years ago." To me, this revelation was incredible—it was like a spiritual spark igniting within me. For the first time, I felt deeply connected to all forms of life. This beautiful, intricate energy that started from a single cell over 2.5 billion years ago has carried a core mission: survival. From that single cell, life expanded into the extraordinary diversity we see today, including us—conscious, thinking, multicellular organisms that make up the human experience.

At its core, life on this planet is about survival. And as a species, we have evolved not only to survive but to heal. Healing is an intrinsic part of our survival mechanism. I begin this book with this understanding because I want you to feel comforted, knowing that you carry 4 billion years of evolutionary wisdom within you. You see it in action every time you get a cut or a scrape, and your body naturally heals itself over time.

One particularly memorable example of this occurred about ten years ago when I was referred to a ninety-three-year-old patient who had a type of facial cancer called Merkel Cell Carcinoma. This cancer is highly aggressive and required a large excision. However, due to her advanced age and multiple underlying medical conditions, I couldn't perform major reconstructive surgery. I had to leave her with a large, three-inch wound over her left cheek. Every week, she came in for a follow-up, and I cleaned and changed her bandage. What amazed me was that, over the course of eight months, her skin completely healed. Week by week, the wound became smaller until it finally closed. The human body is truly miraculous.

The complex processes that drive healing are coded in our DNA. This understanding should give you some comfort, especially if you're facing surgery or recovering from an injury. You are supported by millions of years of evolution and an intricate biological system designed to repair and heal. For the sake of completeness, I'll now describe the four phases of healing. Understanding these phases is important because in the following chapters, I'll explain how you can support your body's healing journey through proper nutrition and diet.

Understanding the Body's Healing Process

When you undergo surgery or experience an injury, your body embarks on a complex healing journey. Understanding this process will help you appreciate why proper nutrition is crucial for recovery. While some aspects of healing may sound a bit scientific, I've kept the explanations as simple as possible so that you'll feel empowered to take control of your healing process. You can think of surgery as a controlled, planned injury. Armed with this foundational knowledge, you'll be well-prepared for what lies ahead—whether before surgery, during recovery, or even in the event of an unexpected injury.

The Four Phases of Healing

1. Hemostasis (Immediate to a Few Minutes Post-Injury)

- **TIMELINE:** Starts immediately after your injury and lasts a few minutes.
  - → Hemostasis is your body's immediate response to an injury, with the goal of stopping the bleeding. As soon as damage occurs, your body activates its blood clotting system to form a barrier that prevents further blood loss. Platelets—specialized blood cells—are drawn to the site, where they become sticky upon contact with collagen in the damaged tissue. This triggers the formation of a clot as the enzyme thrombin creates a mesh of fibrin (a protein) that holds the platelets together. In surgery, we can control this phase using tools like cautery to stop bleeding instantly. However, in later chapters, we'll discuss supplements and vitamins that should be avoided during this phase to prevent bleeding complications.

2. Inflammatory Phase (0–6 Days Post-Injury)

- **TIMELINE:** Typically lasts from 2 to 6 days after surgery.
  - → If the first phase focuses on stopping blood loss, the second phase—often called the Defensive or Inflammatory Phase—focuses on cleaning up damaged cells and preventing infection. White blood cells, known as neutrophils, are the first responders, rushing to the wound site to clear out bacteria and dead tissue. They are most active during the first 24 to 48 hours and begin to decrease after three days. As neutrophils leave, another type of white blood cell, called macrophages, takes over. Macrophages continue to clean the area and release signals to recruit more immune cells to help repair the tissue. This phase is marked by swelling, redness, warmth, and sometimes pain, but it is a critical part of the healing process.

3. Proliferative Phase (4-24 Days Post-Injury)

- **TIMELINE:** Typically lasts from 4 to 24 days post-injury.
  → Once the wound is clean, the Proliferative Phase begins, focusing on rebuilding the damaged area. During this phase, the body works to fill, contract, and cover the wound. Granulation tissue, which is new connective tissue rich in blood vessels, starts to form. The wound edges contract, pulling the wound together, and epithelial cells spread across the surface to cover it with new skin. This phase is key to closing the wound and restoring tissue integrity.

4. Maturation or Remodeling Phase (21 Days to 2 Years Post-Injury)

- **TIMELINE:** Can last from 21 days up to 2 years, depending on the wound's severity.
  → In the final phase, known as the Maturation or Remodeling Phase, the newly formed tissue is strengthened and refined. Collagen fibers are reorganized to make the tissue more resilient, but it will typically only regain about 80 percent of its original strength. Depending on the injury, this phase can last for months or even years. Although the healing process is complex, and factors like infection or overall health can interfere, your body's ability to repair itself is extraordinary.

This timeline graphic visually represents the progression through the four phases of healing. It helps clarify the duration and importance of each phase, providing a clear foundation for understanding how your body heals.

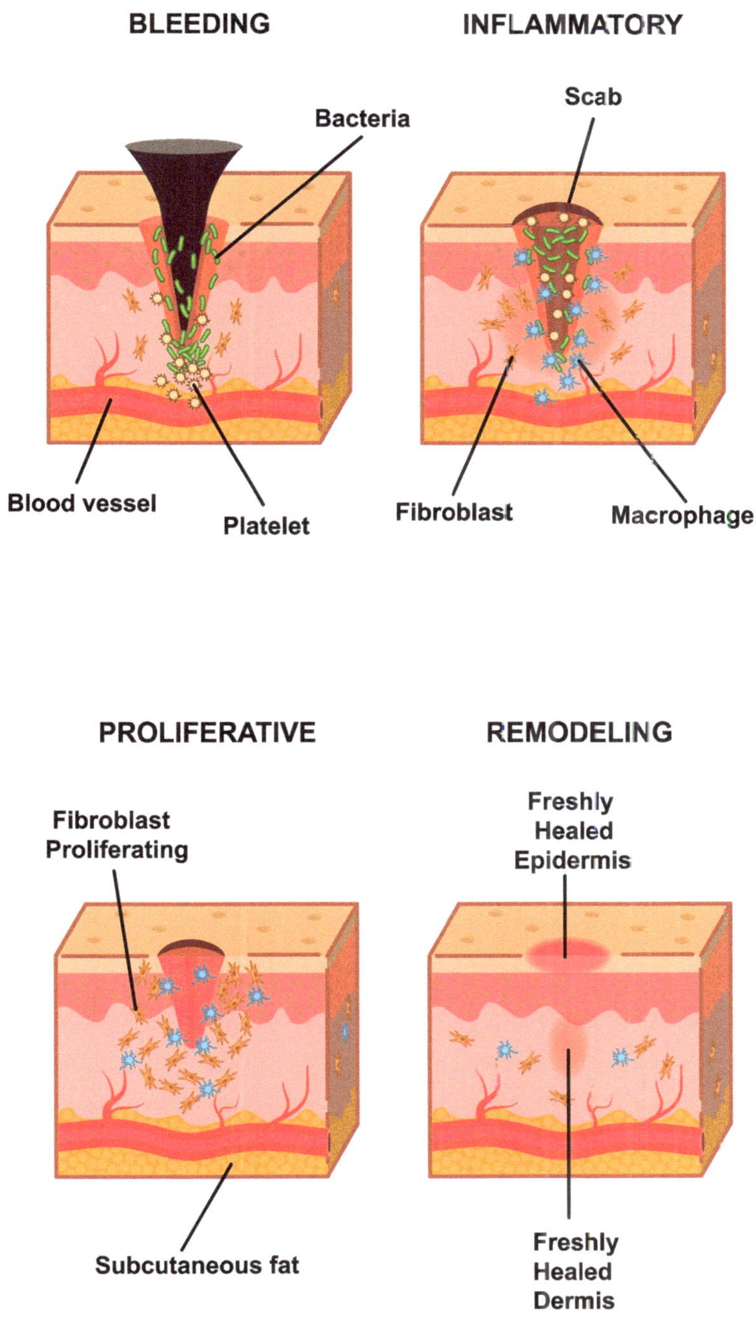
BLEEDING
Bacteria
Blood vessel
Platelet
INFLAMMATORY
Scab
Fibroblast
Macrophage
PROLIFERATIVE
Fibroblast
Proliferating
Subcutaneous fat
REMODELING
Freshly
Healed
Epidermis
Freshly
Healed
Dermis

TAKEAWAY

—

HEALING REQUIRES NUTRIENTS

Your healing journey is a testament to your human body's resilience and the intricate biological processes refined over billions of years. From stopping bleeding to regenerating tissue, your body follows a precise roadmap to recovery, all coded in your DNA. While the body is naturally equipped to heal, its ability to do so efficiently depends on the support you provide.

Healing requires energy, and energy comes from the nutrients you consume. That is where macronutrients and micronutrients—your body's healing fuel—come in. If you understand what you put into your body and how it helps, you will be able to enhance its natural healing abilities. Nutrients provide the foundation upon which your body regenerates and recovers, helping you heal better, faster, and stronger. Let's now look at how these essential nutrients work in the next chapter.

2

The Building Blocks of Healing: Understanding Macronutrients & Micronutrients

The Sacred Dance of Life and Nutrients

Imagine, for a moment, taking a bite of a crisp, juicy apple. As you savor its sweetness, pause to consider the profound journey that brought this simple fruit, and all its nourishing elements, to your plate. The nutrients packed within that apple are not merely fuel for your body; they are the embodiment of a deep, historic relationship between you and the earth, a bond that has taken billions of years to evolve.

When you consume that apple, you're not just eating food. You're participating in an ancient, sacred dance of life—a beautiful, intricate web of co-dependency that connects all living things on our planet. This dance began in the primordial seas billions of years ago and has continued, unbroken, to this very moment.

Consider the glucose in that apple. Its sweet energy is the product of sunlight, captured by the tree's leaves through the miracle of photosynthesis—a process that emerged some 3.4 billion years ago. The vitamins and minerals within the fruit are elements that have existed since the formation of the earth, cycled countless times through rock, soil, and living beings before finding their way into this apple and, ultimately, into you.

This codependency, this interconnectedness, is not just beautiful—it's essential. Life on earth has evolved in such a way that we don't merely need nutrients from other forms of life for energy, but for our very survival. We are not isolated beings, but rather integral parts of a grand, cosmic ecosystem.

The protein you get from a handful of nuts, the omega-3 fatty acids from a piece of fish, the vitamin C from an orange—each of these represents a strand in the intricate tapestry of life. Our bodies have evolved to require these specific nutrients because, over millions of years, we have been in constant dialogue with our environment, adapting to use what was available, and in turn, shaping the world around us.

As we delve deeper into the world of macronutrients and micronutrients in this chapter, I invite you to hold onto this sense of wonder and interconnectedness. When we discuss proteins, carbohydrates, fats, vitamins, and minerals, remember that we're not just talking about abstract biochemical concepts. We're exploring the very language of life on earth—a language that your body speaks fluently, thanks to eons of evolutionary wisdom.

This understanding becomes even more profound when we consider healing. The nutrients we'll discuss are not just passive building blocks, but active participants in your body's incredible ability to repair and regenerate. They carry within them the collective resilience of all life on Earth—a resilience that becomes yours when you nourish yourself mindfully.

So, as we embark on this exploration of nutrients and their roles in healing, let's approach it not just with scientific curiosity, but with a sense of reverence for the intricate dance of life that makes it all possible. By understanding the deep, spiritual connection between the nutrients we consume and our own being, we can approach our diet—and our healing process—with a newfound appreciation and intentionality.

In the sections that follow, we'll break down the various macronutrients and micronutrients, exploring their specific roles in the body and in the healing process. But as we do so, let's keep in mind the bigger picture—the beautiful, cosmic dance that brings these nutrients from the earth, through our food, and into our bodies, where they work their subtle magic to support our health and healing.

Macronutrients vs. Micronutrients: The Big Players and the Vital Supporters

Imagine your body as a bustling city, constantly building, repairing, and maintaining its infrastructure. In this analogy, macronutrients are like the construction materials—the bricks, steel, and concrete needed in large quantities to build and repair structures. Micronutrients, on the other hand, are like specialized tools and skilled workers—smaller in quantity but crucial for ensuring the construction process runs smoothly and efficiently.

Macronutrients: The Building Blocks

Macronutrients, as the name suggests, are nutrients that your body needs in macro (large) amounts. They are the primary sources of energy and the raw materials your body uses to function, grow, and repair itself. The three main categories of macronutrients are:

PROTEINS
CARBOHYDRATES
FATS

These are the nutrients you'll see prominently displayed on food labels, often measured in grams. Your body requires these in relatively large quantities, typically tens or hundreds of grams per day, depending on your size, activity level, and health status.

Micronutrients: The Essential Helpers

Micronutrients, in contrast, are needed in micro (small) amounts. But don't let their small quantities fool you—these nutrients are absolutely essential for your health and healing. Micronutrients include:

VITAMINS
MINERALS
PHYTONUTRIENTS

While you might only need milligrams or even micrograms of these nutrients daily, a deficiency in any of them can significantly impact your health and healing process.

The Synergy of Macro and Micro

It's important to understand that macronutrients and micronutrients don't work in isolation. They have a synergistic relationship, each supporting the functions of the other. For instance:

- **Vitamin D** (a micronutrient) is necessary for the proper absorption of calcium (another micronutrient), which in turn is crucial for protein (a macronutrient) function in muscle contraction and bone formation.
- **B vitamins** (micronutrients) are essential for your body to properly metabolize and use the energy from carbohydrates (macronutrients).

In the context of healing, this synergy becomes even more critical. Your body needs the energy and building blocks provided by macronutrients to carry out repairs, but it also requires the catalytic and regulatory functions of micronutrients to ensure these processes occur efficiently and effectively.

As we delve deeper into each category in the following sections, keep in mind this interconnected nature of nutrients. Understanding this will help you make informed decisions about your diet, ensuring you're providing your body with all the tools it needs to heal optimally.

Remember, in the grand orchestra of healing, macronutrients might be the loud, attention-grabbing instruments, but micronutrients are the conductor, ensuring everything works in harmony. In the next sections, we'll explore each of these nutrient categories in detail, uncovering their specific roles in the healing process.

MACRONUTRIENTS

Required in relatively **larger** amounts.

CARBOHYDRATES

Provide energy support, digestive health, and immune function.

LIPIDS (FATS)

Support cellular function and structure; regulate temperature, protect organs, and store energy in the body.

PROTEIN

Regulate cellular processes, support mechanical and structural functions, and provide energy.

MICRONUTRIENTS

Required in relatively **smaller** amounts.

VITAMINS

Support cell function, development, and growth; function as antioxidants; assist the absorption of other nutrients.

MINERALS

Support bone, muscular, cardiovascular, and nervous system functions; produce enzymes and hormones.

PHYTOCHEMICALS / PHYTONUTRIENTS

Not considered essential; may help prevent chronic diseases and have anti-inflammatory, anti-microbial, and antioxidant effects.

Macronutrients: The Building Blocks of Healing

Now that we understand the distinction between macronutrients and micronutrients, let's zoom in on the macronutrients. As I mentioned, these are the nutrients your body needs in large quantities to fuel the healing process. Remember, they're like the major infrastructure in our city analogy—the foundation upon which all healing is built.

WHY ARE MACRONUTRIENTS IMPORTANT?

- Proteins provide the building blocks for new tissue.
- Carbohydrates supply the energy needed for the repair process.
- Fats support cell formation and regulate the healing response.
- **Energy:** Macronutrients provide the calories needed to fuel the body's recovery processes.
- **Tissue Repair:** Protein plays a direct role in repairing and building new tissue.
- **Inflammation Management:** Healthy fats help reduce inflammation, which is critical during the healing process.

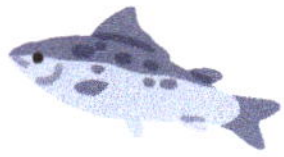

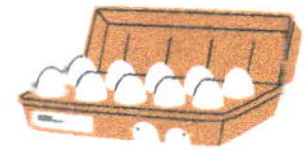

Proteins: The Master Builders

Proteins are often called the building blocks of life, and for good reason. When it comes to healing, proteins are your body's master builders, playing a crucial role in tissue repair and regeneration.

Role in Healing	TISSUE REPAIR	Proteins provide the raw materials for rebuilding damaged tissues. Amino acids, the components of proteins, are used to create new skin, muscle, and other tissues.
	IMMUNE FUNCTION	Many immune system components, including antibodies, are made from proteins. A strong immune system is crucial for preventing infections during the healing process.
	ENZYME PRODUCTION	Proteins form enzymes that catalyze various healing processes, from blood clotting to collagen synthesis.
Protein Sources	ANIMAL SOURCES	Meat, fish, eggs, dairy
	PLANT SOURCES	Beans, lentils, nuts, seeds, soy products
Protein Needs During Healing	During recovery, your protein needs may increase by 20–50 percent depending on the extent of the injury or surgery. For example, if your normal protein intake is 0.8g per kg of body weight, during healing, it might increase to 1.2–1.5g per kg.	

Carbohydrates: The Energy Providers

While often vilified in popular diet culture, carbohydrates play a vital role in the healing process. They are your body's preferred source of energy, and healing is an energy-intensive process.

Role in Healing	ENERGY PRODUCTION	Carbs provide the energy needed for cellular repair and regeneration.
	PROTEIN SPARING	Adequate carb intake prevents the body from breaking down proteins for energy, allowing proteins to focus on tissue repair.
	FIBER FOR GUT HEALTH	Fiber, a type of carbohydrate, supports gut health, which is crucial for overall healing and immune function.
Carbohydrate Sources	COMPLEX CARBS	Whole grains, vegetables, legumes
	SIMPLE CARBS	Fruits, milk, honey
Carbohydrate Needs During Healing	While specific needs vary, generally, carbohydrates should make up about 45–65 percent of your total calorie intake during healing.	

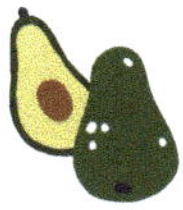

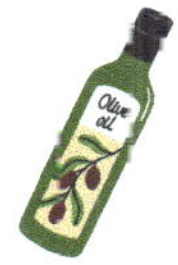

Fats: The Unsung Heroes

Fats have gotten a bad rap, but they're essential for healing as well. They play crucial roles in hormone production, inflammation regulation, and nutrient absorption.

Role in Healing	CELL MEMBRANE FORMATION	Fats are essential components of all cell membranes, including those of new cells formed during healing. They play a key role in cell repair.
	INFLAMMATION REGULATION	Omega-3 fatty acids, in particular, help manage the inflammatory response, which is a crucial part of the healing process.
	HORMONE PRODUCTION	Fats are necessary for the production of hormones that regulate various aspects of healing and metabolism.
	NUTRIENT ABSORPTION	Certain vitamins (A, D, E, K) are fat-soluble, meaning fats are necessary for their absorption.
Fat Sources	HEALTHY FATS	Avocados, nuts, seeds, olive oil, fatty fish
	LIMIT	Saturated and trans fats found in processed foods and some animal products.
Fat Needs During Healing	Fats should typically make up about 20–35 percent of your total calorie intake. Focus on sources of healthy fats, particularly those rich in omega-3 fatty acids.	

MYTH	FACT
High protein intake is always better for healing.	Moderate, balanced protein intake is optimal for most healing processes. While protein is crucial for tissue repair, excessive intake doesn't speed healing and can stress the kidneys. Aim for 1.2–2g per kg of body weight, depending on the extent of healing needed.
All fats should be avoided during healing to reduce inflammation.	Certain fats, especially omega-3s, can actually support the healing process. Healthy fats like those found in fish, nuts, and olive oil can help manage inflammation and support hormone production necessary for healing.
Carbohydrates should be minimized to promote faster healing.	Carbohydrates provide essential energy for the healing process. Complex carbs fuel the energy-intensive process of tissue repair and help spare protein for rebuilding rather than energy production.
You need to dramatically increase calorie intake when healing.	A moderate increase in calories is usually sufficient. While healing does require energy, dramatic increases aren't typically necessary. Focus on nutrient-dense foods rather than just increasing calories.
Plant-based diets can't provide enough protein for healing.	Well-planned plant-based diets can meet protein needs for healing. Combinations of legumes, grains, nuts, and seeds can provide all essential amino acids needed for tissue repair.
Eating extra protein will automatically build more muscle during recovery.	Protein intake must be paired with appropriate physical activity for muscle building. While protein provides the building blocks, muscle synthesis also requires proper stimulus through exercise or physical therapy.
Sugar intake should be completely eliminated during healing.	Small amounts of simple sugars can be part of a balanced healing diet. While excessive sugar can impair healing, moderate amounts in whole fruits can provide quick energy and beneficial micronutrients.
Timing of macronutrient intake doesn't matter for healing.	Strategic timing of nutrients can optimize the healing process. For example, consuming protein shortly after physical therapy can support muscle repair and growth.

Remember, individual nutritional needs during healing can vary based on factors such as age, the extent of the injury or surgery, overall health status, and specific medical conditions. Always consult with a healthcare professional or registered dietitian for personalized advice on optimizing your macronutrient intake for healing.

Balancing Act: The Macronutrient Trio in Healing

While we've discussed each macronutrient separately, it's crucial to understand that they work synergistically in the healing process. A balanced intake of all three is key to optimal healing.

Consider this: If you focus solely on protein intake but neglect carbohydrates, your body might end up breaking down that precious protein for energy instead of using it for tissue repair. Similarly, without adequate fat intake, your body might struggle to manage inflammation effectively, potentially slowing the healing process.

We will discuss this in more detail in later chapters. As you plan your meals during recovery, aim for a balance of all three macronutrients. A typical plate might include a portion of lean protein (like chicken or tofu), a serving of complex carbohydrates (such as brown rice or sweet potato), and a source of healthy fats (like avocado or olive oil), along with plenty of vegetables for additional nutrients and fiber.

Remember, the specific balance of macronutrients can vary based on individual factors like age, sex, activity level, and the nature of the injury or surgery. Always consult with your healthcare provider or a registered dietitian for personalized advice.

In the next section, we'll explore how micronutrients complement these macronutrients, working together to orchestrate the complex symphony of healing in your body.

Micronutrients: The Vital Catalysts of Healing

While macronutrients provide the energy and building blocks for healing, micronutrients act as the vital catalysts that enable and optimize the healing process. These nutrients, needed in smaller quantities but no less important, include vitamins, minerals, and phytonutrients. Let's explore how these micronutrients contribute to your body's healing capabilities.

Vitamins: The Biochemical Facilitators

Vitamins are organic compounds that play crucial roles in various aspects of healing. But have you ever wondered how these essential micronutrients became part of our diet? Let's take a brief journey through evolutionary history to understand the origins of vitamins and their integration into the food chain.

The Evolutionary Tale of Vitamins

Billions of years ago, in the primordial soup of early earth, simple organic molecules began to form more complex structures. Among these were the precursors to what we now know as vitamins. As life evolved, these compounds became integral to various biochemical processes.

EARLY AUTOTROPHS: The first living organisms, such as certain bacteria and algae, could synthesize all the organic compounds they needed, including vitamin-like molecules.

EVOLUTION OF HETEROTROPHS: As more complex organisms evolved, some lost the ability to synthesize certain compounds, including some vitamins. These organisms had to obtain these essential molecules from their environment or diet.

SYMBIOTIC RELATIONSHIPS: Some animals developed symbiotic relationships with microorganisms that could produce vitamins. For example, ruminants like cows have gut bacteria that produce vitamin K and B vitamins.

DIETARY ADAPTATIONS: As species evolved to occupy different niches, their diets changed, leading to varying abilities to synthesize or store different vitamins. For instance, most mammals can synthesize vitamin C, but primates (including humans) lost this ability millions of years ago. That's why we need to get our vitamin C from fruits and vegetables.

This evolutionary history explains why different species have different vitamin requirements and why we need to obtain certain vitamins from our diet.

WHY ARE VITAMINS IMPORTANT?

Vitamins are critical for maintaining your energy levels, supporting your immune health, and aiding in the repair of your tissues. During recovery, vitamins help reduce inflammation, promote wound healing, and replenish energy stores.

Types of Vitamins

Fat-Soluble Vitamins

VITAMINS A D E K

- These vitamins dissolve in dietary fats and can be stored in the body for long periods, mainly in the liver and fat tissues.
- Generally they don't need to be consumed daily.
- Because they are stored, it's important not to consume too much, as excess can be toxic.

VITAMIN	ROLE	NATURAL SOURCES
A 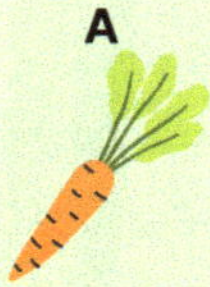	This vitamin is necessary for skin and tissue repair, and it also supports immune function, ensuring your body can ward off infections during the vulnerable post-surgery period.	Carrots, sweet potatoes, leafy greens, liver, and egg yolks.
D 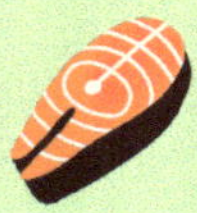	Essential for immune system function and bone healing, Vitamin D helps your body absorb calcium more effectively, promoting faster recovery for surgeries involving bones or joints. Adequate levels of Vitamin D also reduce inflammation and the risk of infections post-surgery.	Sunlight, fatty fish (salmon, tuna), fortified milk, and egg yolks.
E 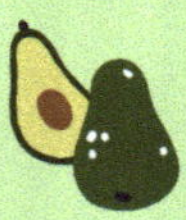	As a potent antioxidant, Vitamin E helps protect your cells from oxidative stress, which can occur during the healing process. It also supports skin healing and reduces scarring.	Nuts (almonds, sunflower seeds), spinach, and avocado.
K 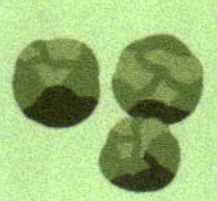	Crucial for blood clotting and bone metabolism, making it important for preventing excessive bleeding during surgery recovery.	Leafy green vegetables (kale, spinach), broccoli, and Brussels sprouts.

Water-Soluble Vitamins

VITAMINS C AND Bs

- These vitamins dissolve in water and are not stored in the body, meaning they must be consumed regularly.
- They are easily absorbed into the bloodstream.
- They are not stored in large amounts (except B12).
- Excess amounts are usually excreted in urine.

VITAMIN	CHARACTERISTICS	NATURAL SOURCES
C 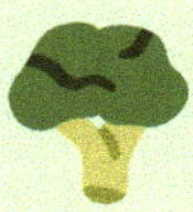	This vitamin is indispensable for collagen production, which plays a crucial role in wound healing and skin repair. Collagen is the protein that holds the skin, muscles, and other tissues together. Additionally, Vitamin C's antioxidant properties protect cells from oxidative stress and inflammation, ensuring faster recovery.	Citrus fruits (oranges, lemons), strawberries, bell peppers, and broccoli.
B	This group of vitamins plays crucial roles in energy production, cell metabolism, and overall tissue repair. Let's break down each subtype. (B1, B2, B3, B5, B6, B7, B9, B12)	A variety of foods broken down in the next column.

Detailed Breakdown of B Vitamins

VITAMIN	FUNCTION	NATURAL SOURCES	IMPORTANCE IN RECOVERY
B1 (Thiamine) 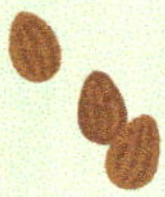	Essential for energy production, especially from carbohydrates. It helps convert carbohydrates into glucose, which the body uses for energy. Thiamine also supports nerve function.	Whole grains, pork, legumes, and nuts.	Thiamine helps the body efficiently use energy during recovery, which is critical for healing and rebuilding tissue.
B2 (Riboflavin) 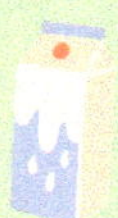	Plays a role in energy production and the breakdown of fats, proteins, and carbohydrates. Riboflavin is also important for skin health and maintaining healthy mucous membranes.	Eggs, dairy products, lean meats, green vegetables, and almonds.	Helps repair damaged tissue and promotes healthy skin, making it important for wound healing.
B3 (Niacin) 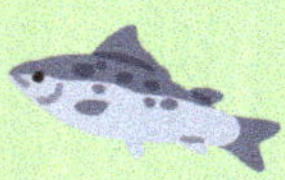	Involved in over 200 enzymatic reactions, niacin helps convert food into energy and plays a role in DNA repair and the stress response.	Meat, poultry, fish, fortified cereals, and legumes.	Niacin improves circulation and helps reduce inflammation, both of which are vital during recovery.
B5 (Pantothenic Acid) 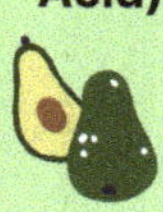	Required for the synthesis of coenzyme A, which is important for fatty acid metabolism. It also supports the production of hormones and cholesterol.	Avocados, eggs, mushrooms, chicken, and sweet potatoes.	Pantothenic acid is necessary for cellular repair and energy production during the healing process.

B6 (Pyridoxine) 	Helps the body convert proteins and glycogen into energy. It is also involved in the production of neurotransmitters and hemoglobin.	Fish, beef liver, potatoes, and bananas.	B6 supports immune function and helps the body produce the red blood cells needed for oxygen transport during recovery.
B7 (Biotin) 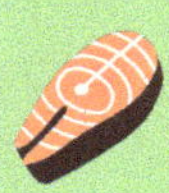	Known for its role in maintaining healthy hair, skin, and nails. Biotin is also involved in the metabolism of fatty acids, amino acids, and glucose.	Eggs, salmon, nuts, seeds, and sweet potatoes.	Biotin aids in tissue repair and cellular regeneration, which are essential for post-surgery recovery.
B9 (Folate or Folic Acid) 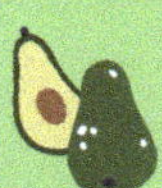	Critical for DNA synthesis and repair, as well as red blood cell production. It also supports tissue growth and proper cell division.	Leafy greens, asparagus, avocados, and beans.	Folate aids in tissue regeneration and supports immune function, helping the body recover faster.
B12 (Cobalamin) 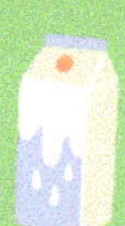	Vital for nerve function, the production of red blood cells, and DNA synthesis. B12 also plays a role in preventing anemia, which can hinder recovery.	Meat, fish, dairy products, and fortified cereals.	B12 helps the body produce the red blood cells needed to transport oxygen to healing tissues, making it essential for recovery.

Key Vitamins for Healing

VITAMIN	ROLE	NATURAL SOURCES
C	Essential for collagen synthesis, a critical component of wound healing	Citrus fruits, berries, bell peppers, broccoli
A	Supports cell differentiation and immune function. Promotes the formation of new skin cells and supports immune response.	Sweet potatoes, carrots, spinach, eggs.
E	Powerful antioxidant that protects cells from damage. Reduces inflammation and supports skin health.	Nuts, seeds, avocados, vegetable oils.
D	Regulates calcium absorption and immune function. Supports bone healing and modulates immune response.	Sunlight exposure, fatty fish, fortified foods.
B-Complex	Essential for energy metabolism and nerve function. Supports energy production for healing processes and promotes nerve repair.	Whole grains, legumes, nuts, meat

Minerals: The Structural Supporters

Minerals are inorganic elements that are crucial for the proper functioning of the body. They are involved in forming bones and teeth, regulating muscle and nerve function, and balancing electrolytes. Unlike vitamins, which are organic, minerals come from the earth and enter the food chain through plants and animals.

Types of Minerals

Macrominerals

These are minerals required in larger amounts by the body.

MINERAL	ROLE	NATURAL SOURCES
Calcium	Particularly important if your surgery involves bones or joints, calcium supports bone regeneration and helps maintain muscle function. Also plays a key role in muscle contraction and blood clotting.	Dairy products (milk, cheese, yogurt), fortified plant-based milk, tofu, and broccoli.
Magnesium	Magnesium is involved in over 300 biochemical reactions in the body, including muscle relaxation, energy production, and the repair of tissues. It helps reduce inflammation and prevent post-surgical complications like muscle cramps.	Nuts (almonds, cashews), spinach, whole grains, and legumes.
Potassium	Sodium helps regulate fluid balance and nerve function. It's particularly important for maintaining hydration, especially after surgery, when dehydration can be a concern.	Bananas, potatoes, spinach, avocados, and beans.
Sodium	Sodium is vital for maintaining electrolyte balance, especially after surgery, when dehydration or fluid imbalances can occur. It also supports muscle contractions and nerve impulses, helping with recovery from physical trauma. It helps regulate blood pressure and supports muscle and nerve function. It works closely with potassium to maintain the body's water balance.	Table salt, seafood, beets, celery, and dairy products.
Phosphorus	Works alongside calcium to maintain strong bones and teeth. It also plays a role in energy production and storage.	Meat, dairy, nuts, seeds, and whole grains.

Trace Minerals

Needed in smaller amounts, but still essential.

MINERAL	ROLE	NATURAL SOURCES
Iron 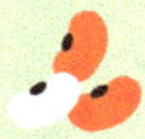	This mineral is essential for producing hemoglobin, the molecule in red blood cells that carries oxygen to tissues. Adequate iron ensures that healing tissues receive sufficient oxygen, speeding up recovery and reducing fatigue.	Red meat, spinach, lentils, fortified cereals, and beans.
Zinc 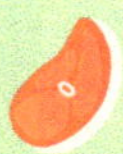	It is vital for wound healing because it supports DNA synthesis, cell division, and protein production—all critical processes for tissue repair. It also bolsters the immune system, reducing the risk of post-surgical infections.	Oysters, beef, chickpeas, pumpkin seeds, and cashews.
Copper 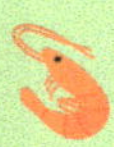	Helps with the absorption of iron and the formation of red blood cells. It also supports connective tissue health.	Shellfish, nuts, seeds, and whole grains.
Selenium 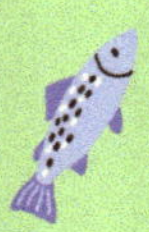	Acts as a potent antioxidant, protecting cells from damage and supporting thyroid function.	Brazil nuts, fish, eggs, and sunflower seeds.

Key Minerals for Healing

MINERAL	ROLE	NATURAL SOURCES	HEALING IMPACT
Zinc	Essential for protein synthesis and immune function.	Oysters, beef, pumpkin seeds, lentils.	Accelerates wound healing and supports immune response.
Iron	Crucial for oxygen transport in the blood.	Red meat, spinach, and lentils.	Supports tissue oxygenation and energy production.
Calcium	Essential for bone formation and muscle function.	Dairy products, leafy greens, fortified plant milks.	Critical for bone healing and muscle repair.
Magnesium	Involved in over three hundred enzymatic reactions in the body.	Nuts, seeds, whole grains, leafy greens.	Supports energy production and muscle and nerve function.

Phytonutrients: Nature's Healing Boosters

Phytonutrients, also known as phytochemicals, are naturally occurring compounds found in plants. Although they are not considered essential nutrients like vitamins and minerals, phytochemicals offer numerous health benefits. They provide plants with color, flavor, and resistance to disease, and when consumed, they protect the body from oxidative stress, inflammation, and cellular damage, making them particularly beneficial during the healing process.

Types of Phytochemicals

PHYTOCHEMICALS	ROLE	NATURAL SOURCES
Flavonoids 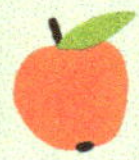	These compounds are known for their antioxidant properties and their role in improving heart health, reducing inflammation, and supporting immune function.	Berries, apples, onions, green tea, and citrus fruits.
Carotenoid 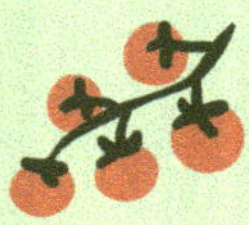	These pigments provide the red, orange, and yellow colors in fruits and vegetables. Carotenoids are powerful antioxidants that can be converted into vitamin A in the body.	Carrots, sweet potatoes, tomatoes, and leafy greens like spinach.
Polyphenols 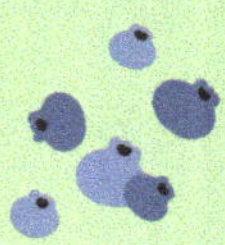	Known for their anti-inflammatory and antioxidant properties, polyphenols help protect against cardiovascular diseases and reduce oxidative stress in the body.	Green tea, red wine, dark chocolate, grapes, and berries.
Saponins 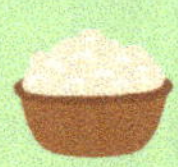	These compounds have immune-boosting properties and help regulate cholesterol levels.	Legumes such as beans, lentils, soy, and oats.
Sulforaphane 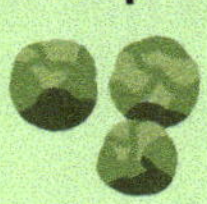	A sulfur-rich compound that stimulates the body's detoxification enzymes and has been shown to have anti-cancer properties.	Cruciferous vegetables like broccoli, Brussels sprouts, and cauliflower.

Key Phytonutrients for Healing

PHYTONUTRIENTS	ROLE	NATURAL SOURCES
Flavonoids 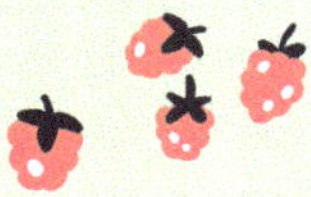	Powerful antioxidants with anti-inflammatory properties. Reduce inflammation and oxidative stress.	Berries, tea, citrus fruits, dark chocolate
Carotenoids 	Precursors to Vitamin A and potent antioxidants. Support immune function and protect cells from damage.	Orange and red fruits and vegetables
Glucosinolates 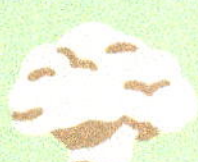	Support detoxification processes. Enhance the body's ability to remove toxins, supporting overall healing.	Cruciferous vegetables like broccoli, cauliflower, and Brussels sprouts

WHY ARE PHYTONUTRIENTS IMPORTANT?

Phytonutrients, though not classified as essential nutrients, play a critical role in protecting the body from oxidative damage, reducing inflammation, and supporting immune function. They help the body recover more effectively by promoting tissue repair and reducing the risk of infection during recovery.

The Micronutrient Symphony in Healing

Just as an orchestra requires all instruments playing in harmony to create beautiful music, your body needs a full complement of micronutrients working together to orchestrate optimal healing. For example:

- **VITAMIN C** works synergistically with iron to enhance its absorption, ensuring adequate oxygen supply to healing tissues. Vitamin C needs can double or triple during wound healing.
- **IRON** needs may rise to support increased blood production and tissue oxygenation.
- **VITAMIN D** partners with calcium for proper bone healing and immune function.
- **ZINC** collaborates with vitamin A to support skin healing and immune response. Zinc requirements may increase by 50 percent following surgery or injury.

Understanding these interactions underscores the importance of a varied, nutrient-rich diet during healing. Focusing on a single "superfood" or nutrient is less effective than consuming a diverse range of whole foods that provide a spectrum of micronutrients. In later chapters, we'll explore how to practically incorporate these macro and micronutrients into your diet to support optimal healing.

MYTH	FACT
If some vitamins are good, more is always better.	Excessive intake of certain vitamins and minerals can be harmful. For example, too much vitamin A can actually impair wound healing and cause other health issues.
All your micronutrient needs can be met with a multivitamin supplement.	While supplements can be helpful in some cases, they don't provide the full spectrum of nutrients found in whole foods. A varied diet is usually the best way to meet micronutrient needs.
Vitamin C is the only important vitamin for wound healing.	While vitamin C is crucial, many other vitamins and minerals play important roles. For example, vitamin A, vitamin E, and zinc are also vital for optimal wound healing.
You don't need to worry about micronutrients if you're eating enough calories.	Calorie intake doesn't guarantee proper micronutrient intake. It's possible to consume enough calories but still be deficient in certain vitamins or minerals if your diet isn't varied and nutrient-dense.
Cooking vegetables destroys all their micronutrients.	While some nutrients can be lost in cooking, others actually become more bioavailable. For example, cooking tomatoes increases the availability of lycopene, an important antioxidant.
All phytonutrients are antioxidants.	While many phytonutrients have antioxidant properties, they can have various other functions too, such as modulating immune response or supporting detoxification processes.

TAKEAWAY

—

THE NUTRIENT FOUNDATION FOR HEALING

As we've explored in this chapter, both macronutrients and micronutrients play crucial roles in the complex process of healing. From proteins that provide the building blocks for tissue repair to vitamins and minerals that catalyze essential biochemical reactions, each nutrient contributes to your body's remarkable ability to recover and regenerate. Remember, the key takeaways from this chapter are:

- Macronutrients (proteins, carbohydrates, and fats) provide the energy and raw materials needed for healing.
- Micronutrients (vitamins, minerals, and phytonutrients) act as essential catalysts and regulators in the healing process.
- A balanced, varied diet is typically the best way to ensure you're getting all the nutrients your body needs for optimal healing.
- Individual nutritional needs can vary based on factors like age, the extent of injury or surgery, and overall health status.

By understanding the roles of these nutrients, you're better equipped to make informed decisions about your diet during recovery. However, knowing what your body needs is only part of the equation. In our modern world, actually obtaining these nutrients can be more challenging than you might think.

While we've discussed the importance of various nutrients for healing, you might be wondering, "If I'm eating a typical modern diet, aren't I getting all these nutrients already?" The answer, unfortunately, is not always straightforward.

In the next chapter, we'll explore how changes in food production, processing, and consumption patterns have affected the nutritional quality of our diets. We'll uncover some surprising truths about:

- How modern agricultural practices have impacted the nutrient content of our foods
- The effects of food processing on nutrient availability
- Hidden sources of inflammation in common foods that could be hindering your healing process
- The potential impacts of common dietary patterns on your body's ability to heal

So, let's turn the page and dive into the often-overlooked aspects of our modern diet that could be silently impacting your health and healing potential. Armed with this knowledge, you'll be even better equipped to make choices that support your body's incredible capacity for healing.

3

The Hidden Dangers in Modern Diets

The Evolving Landscape of Our Food

As we journey through the intricate world of nutrition and healing, we find ourselves at a curious crossroads. On one hand, we have unprecedented access to a vast array of foods from around the globe, available at our fingertips year-round. On the other hand, we face a silent crisis in the very foundation of our nourishment.

Imagine, for a moment, your great-grandparents walking into a modern supermarket. They would likely be awestruck by the abundance and variety, yet puzzled by many of the items on the shelves. The truth is, in just a few generations, our food landscape has undergone a radical transformation—one that our bodies are still struggling to adapt to.

This chapter peels back the glossy veneer of modern food to reveal some uncomfortable truths. We'll explore how the quest for efficiency, shelf-life, and profit in our food system has introduced a plethora of chemicals never before encountered by the human body. From artificial preservatives to synthetic food dyes, these novel compounds pose potential risks that we're only beginning to understand.

But the changes go beyond just additives. Modern agricultural practices, while boosting yields, have fundamentally altered the nutrient profiles of our crops. The soil that once teemed with minerals and microorganisms has been depleted, leading to foods that may look the same but offer less nutritional value than their historical counterparts.

Perhaps most alarmingly, we'll uncover how what's considered safe for consumption can vary dramatically depending on where you live. The stark contrast between food regulations in Europe and the United States paints a troubling picture. Ingredients banned across the Atlantic for potential health risks continue to find their way into American foods, raising questions about the adequacy of our regulatory systems.

As we navigate this complex landscape, remember: knowledge is power. Understanding these hidden dangers is the first step towards making informed choices that support your body's innate healing abilities. In the pages that follow, we'll arm you with the insights needed to navigate the modern food maze, empowering you to nourish your body effectively on its journey to recovery.

So, let's embark on this eye-opening exploration of our modern diet—not with fear, but with the curiosity and determination to uncover the truth about what we're really putting on our plates.

The Impact of Modern Agriculture on Nutrient Content

The face of agriculture has changed dramatically over the past century. While these changes have led to increased crop yields and food availability, they've also had profound effects on the nutritional quality of our food. Let's explore some of the key ways modern agricultural practices have impacted the nutrient content of our crops.

Soil Depletion and Nutrient Density

One of the most significant, yet often overlooked, consequences of modern farming practices is soil depletion. Intensive farming, which often involves growing the same crops on the same land year after year, can strip the soil of its natural nutrients. Here are some troubling facts to come to terms with:

- Minerals like iron, zinc, and magnesium, which plants absorb from the soil, have declined in many fruits and vegetables over the past fifty to seventy years.
- A landmark study published in the Journal of the American College of Nutrition compared USDA nutrient content data for forty-three different vegetables and fruits from 1950 and 1999. The study found

significant reductions in the levels of protein, calcium, phosphorus, iron, riboflavin (vitamin B2) and ascorbic acid (vitamin C).

This means that an apple you eat today may have less nutritional value than one your grandparents ate, even if it looks identical.

Monoculture Farming and Reduced Crop Diversity

Modern agriculture often relies on monoculture—the practice of growing a single crop over a large area. While this approach increases efficiency, it comes with several drawbacks:

- Reduced biodiversity in our diets, limiting the range of nutrients we consume.
- Increased vulnerability to pests and diseases, leading to greater reliance on pesticides.
- Soil degradation, as different crops extract and return different nutrients to the soil.

Genetic Modification and Its Potential Impacts

Genetically Modified Organisms (GMOs) have become increasingly common in our food supply. While GMOs can offer benefits like increased yield and pest resistance, their long-term impact on nutrient content and human health is still a subject of debate:

- Studies have found that genetic modifications can lead to decreases in certain micronutrients or increases in antinutrients, which inhibit nutrient absorption. For instance, while enhancing traits like pest resistance or herbicide tolerance, nutrient concentrations like zinc and iron in genetically modified (GM) crops have sometimes shown unintended decreases, impacting the crop's overall nutritional quality.
- There are concerns about the potential for GMOs to introduce new allergens or toxins into the food supply. A well-known case involving

GM soybeans in the 1990s highlighted the risk of introducing allergens. Researchers found that transferring a Brazil nut protein into soybeans (to improve its amino acid profile) created a risk of allergic reactions, prompting them to halt the project. This case demonstrated the importance of allergen testing before GMO release, as some proteins could provoke unexpected allergic responses in sensitive individuals. Regulatory bodies now mandate rigorous allergenicity assessments for all GMOs before approval.

Pesticides, Herbicides, and Their Effects on Nutrient Profiles

The widespread use of chemical pesticides and herbicides in modern farming has implications beyond just killing pests:

- Some pesticides can interfere with plants' abilities to absorb nutrients from the soil.
- Residues from these chemicals on our food may impact our gut microbiome, potentially affecting our ability to absorb nutrients.
- Glyphosate, a common herbicide, has been shown to chelate (bind to) important minerals in the soil, potentially making them less available to plants.

Food Processing and Nutrient Availability

In our modern world, much of the food we consume undergoes significant processing before it reaches our plates. While food processing can offer benefits like improved food safety and extended shelf life, it can also have profound effects on the nutrient content of our food. So, what does this mean for your health?

Common Processing Methods and Their Impact on Nutrients

METHOD	PROS	CONS
Heat Treatment (Cooking, Pasteurization, Sterilization)	Improves food safety, can increase the bioavailability of some nutrients (e.g., lycopene in tomatoes).	Can degrade heat-sensitive vitamins like vitamin C and some B vitamins.
Refining	Increases shelf life and improves texture and appearance of some products.	Removes fiber, essential fatty acids, and many vitamins and minerals.
Freezing	Can preserve nutrients effectively if done quickly after harvest.	Some nutrients may be lost during blanching before freezing.
Canning	Long shelf life, can preserve many nutrients effectively.	Heat-sensitive vitamins may be degraded during the canning process.

Additives and Preservatives: Necessary Evils or Hidden Dangers?

Food additives serve various purposes, from preserving freshness to enhancing flavor. However, some may have unintended health consequences:

- Artificial colors: Some have been linked to behavioral issues in children.
- Preservatives: While they prevent spoilage, some (like nitrites in processed meats) have been associated with increased cancer risk.
- Emulsifiers: Common in processed foods, some studies suggest they may disrupt gut bacteria and promote inflammation.

Fortification: Addressing or Masking Nutritional Deficits?

Food fortification has been used to address widespread nutrient deficiencies:

- **Pros:** Can help prevent deficiencies on a population level (e.g., folic acid in bread to prevent neural tube defects).
- **Cons:** May give a false sense of nutritional adequacy to processed foods, potentially discouraging consumption of naturally nutrient-rich whole foods.

The Rise of Ultra-Processed Foods and Health Implications

Ultra-processed foods now make up a significant portion of many people's diets, especially in western countries:

- Typically high in added sugars, unhealthy fats, and salt.
- Often low in fiber, vitamins, and minerals.
- Associated with increased risk of obesity, type 2 diabetes, and cardiovascular disease.
- May contain higher levels of potentially harmful additives and compounds formed during processing.

Hidden Sources of Inflammation in Common Foods

Inflammation is a natural part of the body's healing process. However, chronic, low-grade inflammation can hinder recovery and contribute to various health issues. Many common foods in the modern diet can promote inflammation, often in ways that aren't immediately obvious. Let's explore some of these hidden sources of inflammation.

Artificial Additives and Their Inflammatory Potential

- **Artificial Sweeteners:**
  - → Despite being calorie-free, some artificial sweeteners may disrupt gut bacteria and potentially trigger inflammatory responses.
  - → Examples: Aspartame, sucralose, saccharin.

- **Artificial Colors and Flavors:**
  - → Some synthetic food dyes have been linked to increased inflammation and behavioral issues, particularly in children.
  - → Examples: Red 40, Yellow 5, Yellow 6.

- **Emulsifiers:**
  - → Common in processed foods, some emulsifiers may alter gut bacteria and intestinal mucus, potentially promoting inflammation.
  - → Examples: Carrageenan, polysorbate 80.

Omega-6 to Omega-3 Imbalance in Modern Diets

- While both omega-6 and omega-3 fatty acids are essential, the modern Western diet often contains an excess of omega-6.
- A high omega-6 to omega-3 ratio can promote inflammation in the body.
- Common sources of excess omega-6: Vegetable oils (soybean, corn, sunflower), processed snack foods.

Gluten and Other Common Food Sensitivities

- For some individuals, gluten can trigger inflammation, even without celiac disease (non-celiac gluten sensitivity).
- Other common inflammatory triggers include dairy, soy, and eggs, though individual responses vary.
- The rise in food sensitivities may be partly due to changes in food processing and agricultural practices.

Advanced Glycation End Products (AGEs) in Processed Foods

- AGEs are harmful compounds formed when proteins or fats combine with sugars (glycation).
- They are naturally produced in the body but are also present in foods, especially those that are highly processed or cooked at high temperatures.
- High levels of dietary AGEs can promote inflammation and oxidative stress.
- Common sources: Fried foods, pasteurized dairy products, processed meats.

Hidden Sugars and Refined Carbohydrates

- Excess sugar consumption can lead to chronic inflammation.
- Many processed foods contain hidden sugars, often under less recognizable names (e.g., dextrose, maltose, rice syrup).
- Refined carbohydrates (white bread, pasta) can spike blood sugar, potentially promoting inflammation.

Trans Fats and Hydrogenated Oils

- Although being phased out, trans fats are still present in some processed foods and are highly inflammatory.
- Even small amounts of trans fats can have negative health effects.
- Look out for "partially hydrogenated oils" on ingredient lists.

The US-Europe Food Regulation Divide: A Shocking Reality Check

Imagine walking into a grocery store and filling your cart with everyday items: a box of Trix cereal for the kids, some Mountain Dew for a party, and a loaf of bread for sandwiches. Now, picture yourself teleporting to a similar store in Paris or Berlin with the same shopping list. You'd be in for a surprise—many of these common American products either wouldn't exist on European shelves or would look dramatically different. Why? Because they contain ingredients that are banned or heavily restricted in the European Union.

The Colorful Deception: A Tale of Two Cereals

Let's start with that box of Trix cereal. In the US, it's a rainbow of vibrant colors, achieved through the use of artificial food dyes like Red 40, Yellow 5, and Blue 1. Now, here's where things get interesting:

- **In the EU:** These artificial colors are required to carry a warning label stating they "may have an adverse effect on activity and attention in children."
- **In the US:** No such warning exists, and these dyes are used liberally in products marketed directly to children.

But it gets even more bizarre. General Mills, the maker of Trix, sells the same cereal in the UK and other European countries. The difference? They use natural colorings derived from fruits and vegetables. The question that should be on every American parent's mind is: If it's possible to make Trix without potentially harmful artificial colors, why isn't this version sold in the US?

The Soda Shocker: Mountain Dew's Secret Ingredient

Grab a bottle of Mountain Dew in the US, and you'll be consuming an ingredient called brominated vegetable oil (BVO). This additive, used to keep the citrus flavoring from separating, is banned in the EU and over one hundred other countries. Why? It contains bromine, an element found in flame retardants, which can build up in the body and potentially lead to memory loss and skin problems.

- **In the EU:** BVO is a no-go. Soft drinks are formulated without it.
- **In the US:** It's still used in citrus-flavored sodas, including some flavors of Gatorade and Powerade.

The most mind-boggling part? PepsiCo, Mountain Dew's parent company, manages to produce BVO-free versions for European markets. Again, we must ask: If it's possible to make these drinks without BVO, why continue to use it in American products?

The Bread Dilemma: Hidden Chemicals in Your Sandwich

That loaf of bread you picked up might contain potassium bromate or azodicarbonamide. These additives, used to strengthen dough and make it rise better, are banned in the EU due to links to cancer and respiratory issues.

- **In the EU:** Bakers use alternatives that don't carry the same health risks.
- **In the US:** These additives are still common in many commercial bread products.

How Is This Possible?

The stark contrast between US and EU regulations on food additives raises serious questions:

1. **Different Philosophies:** The EU operates on a precautionary principle—if there's a suspected risk of harm from an additive, it's restricted or banned until proven safe. The US FDA, however, often allows additives unless they're proven harmful.
2. **Lobbying Power:** The food industry in the US has significant lobbying power, which can influence regulatory decisions.

3. **Consumer Awareness:** European consumers have generally been more vocal about food additives, pushing for stricter regulations.
4. **Regulatory Inertia:** Changing existing regulations in the US is a slow and often difficult process.

The Bottom Line

The fact that major food companies can and do produce safer versions of their products for European markets is perhaps the most damning evidence of all. It proves that removing these controversial ingredients is possible and economically viable.

As American consumers, we're left with a troubling question: Why are we being sold foods with ingredients deemed too risky for consumers in other developed nations? The divide between US and European food regulations isn't just a matter of policy—it's a matter of public health and consumer rights.

Being aware of these differences empowers us to make more informed choices about our food. It also raises important questions about the standards we should expect from our food industry and regulatory bodies. After all, if it's not good enough for Europe, why should it be good enough for us?

On the next page is a list of banned ingredients in Europe (and other countries) that are still permitted in the United States, with an overview of their uses and reasons for their bans.

INGREDIENT	COMMON USE	COUNTRIES BANNING	REASON FOR BAN
Potassium Bromate	Flour treatment agent in bread and baked goods	EU, Canada, Brazil	Classified as a possible human carcinogen; linked to cancer in animal studies and can damage the kidneys and thyroid.
Azodicarbon-amide (ADA)	Flour bleaching and dough conditioner	EU, Australia	Potential respiratory issues upon exposure; breaks down into carcinogenic compounds when baked or heated.
BHA (Butylated Hydroxyanisole)	Preservative in snacks, cereals, and gum	EU, Japan	Potentially carcinogenic, particularly affecting the kidneys; animal studies have linked BHA to cancer.
BHT (Butylated Hydroxytoluene)	Preservative in snacks, cereals, and cosmetics	EU, Japan	Linked to developmental and endocrine effects; suspected to act as a carcinogen and cause allergic reactions in sensitive individuals.

Red Dye #40 (Allura Red AC)	Food coloring in candy, snacks, and beverages	Austria, Norway	Linked to hyperactivity in children; studies suggest potential carcinogenicity and allergy risks.
Yellow Dye #5 (Tartrazine)	Food coloring in beverages, candies, snacks	EU requires labeling, some bans in Norway, Austria	Associated with hyperactivity, allergies, and potential adverse effects on the liver and kidneys.
Yellow Dye #6 (Sunset Yellow FCF)	Food coloring in candies, cereals, baked goods	Norway, Finland	Linked to hyperactivity in children; potential carcinogen and allergy risks.
Ractopamine	Feed additive to promote leanness in meat	EU, Russia, China	Associated with cardiovascular and nervous system issues; banned in animal production due to health concerns for both animals and humans consuming the meat.
Brominated Vegetable Oil (BVO)	Emulsifier in sodas and sports drinks	EU, Japan, India	Linked to neurological symptoms and potential buildup in human tissue; may disrupt thyroid function.

rBGH / rBST (Recombinant Bovine Growth Hormone)	Hormone in dairy production	EU, Canada, Australia	Concerns about increased insulin-like growth factor (IGF-1), which has been linked to cancer risk; animal welfare concerns due to increased health issues in treated cows.
Olestra	Fat substitute in snack foods	UK, Canada	Linked to gastrointestinal distress, depletion of fat-soluble vitamins, and reduced nutrient absorption.
Chlorine-treated Chicken	Antimicrobial in poultry processing	EU	Banned due to concerns about chemical exposure and masking poor hygienic practices in meat processing.
Rhodamine B	Dye for certain foods and cosmetics	EU, China, India	Considered a potential carcinogen with links to liver and kidney damage; banned for use in foods due to health risks.

Navigating the Modern Food Landscape for Optimal Healing

Given the complexities of our modern food system and the regulatory disparities we've discussed, how can we make the best choices for our health, especially when focusing on healing and recovery? Here are some practical strategies to help you navigate this challenging terrain:

1. Prioritize Whole, Minimally Processed Foods

- Focus on fruits, vegetables, whole grains, lean proteins and healthy fats.
- These foods are less likely to contain controversial additives and are generally more nutrient-dense.
- Example: Choose a baked sweet potato over packaged potato chips.

2. Read and Understand Food Labels

- Ingredient list: Ingredients are listed in order of quantity. Be wary of long lists with unfamiliar items.
- Look out for hidden sugars and unhealthy fats.
- Be aware of marketing terms like "natural" which may not have strict regulatory definitions.

3. Choose Organic When Possible

- Prioritize buying organic for the "Dirty Dozen"—produce most likely to have pesticide residues. The 2023 Dirty Dozen list, indicating produce with the highest likelihood of pesticide residues, includes the following items: strawberries, spinach, kale (along with collard and mustard greens), peaches, pears, nectarines, apples, grapes, bell and hot peppers, cherries, blueberries, and green beans. Prioritizing organic options for these items can help reduce exposure to pesticide residues.
- Organic products are less likely to contain synthetic additives and GMOs.
- If budget is a concern, focus on organic for animal products and the most heavily sprayed produce.

4. Opt for Local and Seasonal Foods

- Locally grown produce is often fresher and may retain more nutrients.
- Seasonal eating can provide a natural variety of nutrients throughout the year.
- Consider joining a CSA (Community Supported Agriculture) program for fresh, local produce.

5. Cook More Meals at Home

- This gives you control over ingredients and cooking methods.
- Use herbs and spices for flavor instead of relying on artificial additives.
- Batch cooking can make home-prepared meals more convenient.

6. Stay Hydrated with Clean Water

- Invest in a good water filter if you're concerned about tap water quality.
- Limit sugary drinks and artificial sweeteners.
- Herbal teas can be a good way to increase fluid intake while providing additional health benefits.

7. Consider Supplements Wisely

- While a balanced diet should provide most nutrients, certain supplements may be beneficial during healing.
- Consult with a healthcare professional before starting any supplement regimen.
- Look for third-party tested supplements to ensure quality and purity.

8. Be Mindful of Food Sensitivities

- Pay attention to how different foods make you feel, especially during the healing process.
- Consider keeping a food diary to track any symptoms that may be related to diet.
- Common culprits for sensitivities include dairy, gluten, soy, and eggs.

9. Balance Nutrition with Enjoyment

- Stress and anxiety about food can be counterproductive to healing.
- Allow for occasional treats, focusing on quality over quantity.
- Practice mindful eating to enhance enjoyment and improve digestion.

10. Stay Informed, But Don't Panic

- Keep up with reputable nutrition research, but be wary of fad diets and sensationalized health claims.
- Remember that nutrition science is complex and constantly evolving.
- Focus on long-term patterns rather than obsessing over individual meals or ingredients.

By implementing these strategies, you can navigate the modern food landscape more effectively, making choices that support your body's healing processes. Remember, every small step towards a healthier diet counts. Be patient with yourself as you make these changes, and celebrate the positive choices you make along the way.

4

Proper Nutrition Before & After Surgery

Building a Strong Foundation

Malnutrition doesn't just happen to people who get trapped on a deserted island. If you are not eating mindfully for a consistent period of time, you could be lacking in a score of nutrients. Recent studies have revealed a startling statistic: nearly 50 percent of hospitalized patients are malnourished or at risk of malnutrition before surgery. However, thanks to your investment in yourself by reading this book, you will not be part of this statistic, right?

Modern diets, as discussed in previous chapters, often fall short of providing the essential macronutrients and micronutrients you need to thrive, particularly after surgery. So, let's avoid anything that can slow healing and increase the risk of complications. By incorporating a well-rounded nutritional approach before and after surgery, you can significantly support your body's immune system, reduce inflammation, and promote faster, more efficient healing. Similar to how I healed my finger after I injured it playing catch with my son, you can encourage faster results as well.

QUICK SELF-ASSESSMENT

Before proceeding, assess your current nutritional status:

- Do you eat protein with every meal?
- Do you consume five or more servings of fruits and vegetables daily?
- Do you drink eight or more glasses of water per day?
- Have you maintained a stable weight in the past six months?
- Do you eat a varied diet including different food groups?

Important: If you checked fewer than three boxes, pay special attention to the following guidelines and discuss them with your healthcare provider.

The Power of Nutrition

Proper nutrition serves two primary purposes in surgical preparation and recovery:

a. Enhancing Immunity: Surgery places significant stress on your immune system. A well-nourished body is better equipped to fight off potential infections, a possible risk after surgical procedures. Research has shown that patients with good nutritional status have a lower risk of postoperative infections and complications.

For example, a study found that giving your body nutrients which are known to boost your immune system around the time of surgery reduced postoperative infectious complications by 39 percent in patients undergoing major abdominal surgery. This information may seem obvious, however, you would be surprised how many people still don't prepare by eating such foods. If you can reduce your own risks by more than a third by simply following a nutrient-rich diet, why wouldn't you?

b. Improving Healing: Consuming a variety of key nutrients could help your body with tissue repair and wound healing. Eating a colorful, whole food based diet ensures your body has the necessary building blocks for faster and more effective healing post-surgery.

The impact of proper nutrition on surgical outcomes is profound. If you plan ahead and make sure you get adequate nutrition before and after surgery, you will likely experience:

- A faster recovery time
- A shorter hospital stay
- Fewer postoperative complications
- Improved wound healing
- Better preservation of your muscle mass and strength
- An enhanced overall quality of life during recovery

It's important to note that your nutritional needs can vary based on the type of surgery you're having, your current health status, and other individual factors. I recommend working closely with your healthcare team to develop a personalized nutrition plan for an optimal outcome.

Essential Nutrients

Protein and Amino Acids

You've probably heard the saying, "Your body is a temple." If that's true, then macronutrients are the foundation and structure that hold it together. Without them, your temple would be full of gaps. Among these, protein stands as the cornerstone of post-surgery recovery. It plays a crucial role in rebuilding tissues, maintaining muscle mass, and supporting the production of essential enzymes and hormones—critical components your body needs to heal effectively.

Recommended intake: Current guidelines **suggest 1.2–2.0 grams** per kilogram of body weight per day of protein for surgical patients. This is significantly higher than the 0.8 grams per kilogram of body weight per day recommended for the general population due to the increased demands of healing.

For example, a 70 kg (154 lb) individual preparing for surgery should aim for 84–140 grams of protein per day. This increased protein intake should ideally begin 2–4 weeks before surgery and continue throughout the recovery period.

Best Sources of Protein

- **Lean meats** (chicken, turkey, lean cuts of beef): These provide high-quality complete proteins with all essential amino acids.
- **Fish** (especially fatty fish like salmon, mackerel, and sardines): In addition to protein, these provide omega-3 fatty acids which have anti-inflammatory properties.
- **Eggs**: A complete protein source that's easy to digest and versatile in preparation.
- **Dairy products** (milk, yogurt, cheese): These provide both protein and calcium, which is particularly important for bone health in orthopedic surgeries.
- **Plant-based options** (beans, lentils, tofu, quinoa): These are excellent for those following a vegetarian or vegan diet, or for adding variety to an omnivorous diet.

Best Protein Sources Chart

FOOD	PORTION	PROTEIN (G)	ADDITIONAL BENEFITS
Meat Proteins			
Chicken breast	3 oz	27	Lean protein, B vitamins
Hamburger (80/20)	3 oz	22	Iron, B12, zinc
Pork chop	3 oz	23	Thiamine, phosphorus
Steak (sirloin)	3 oz	26	Iron, B12, zinc
Turkey breast	3 oz	25	Lean protein, selenium

Fish (salmon)	3 oz	22	Omega-3, vitamin D
Fish (tuna)	3 oz	22	Lean protein, selenium
	Dairy & Eggs		
Greek yogurt	1 cup	23	Calcium, probiotics
Cottage cheese	1 cup	24	Calcium, low-fat option
Eggs	2 large	12	Complete protein, vitamin D
	Plant-Based Proteins		
Lentils	1 cup cooked	18	Fiber, iron
Black beans	1 cup cooked	15	Fiber, antioxidants
Chickpeas	1 cup cooked	14	Fiber, magnesium
Edamame	1 cup	17	Fiber, iron
Tempeh	3 oz	16	Probiotics, iron
Tofu (firm)	3 oz	9	Calcium, iron
Quinoa	1 cup cooked	8	Complete protein, fiber
Almonds	¼ cup	7	Healthy fats, vitamin E
Pumpkin seeds	¼ cup	9	Zinc, magnesium

The Role of Amino Acids: Arginine and Glutamine in Surgery Recovery

If you're consuming enough protein from natural sources, you're likely getting a sufficient amount of amino acids, which are naturally found in many types of protein. However, before skipping this section, consider that understanding their role could help optimize your body's healing potential. It's also worth checking whether your intake is truly as optimal as it could be—and, if not, what steps you can take to improve it.

When preparing for or recovering from surgery, your body's nutritional needs go beyond the basics. Two amino acids, arginine and glutamine, play a crucial role in supporting the healing process. Let's explore how these powerful nutrients contribute to recovery, backed by the latest research.

Arginine: The Building Block of Recovery
Arginine is a conditionally essential amino acid, meaning your body can produce it, but during times of stress—like surgery—your needs might exceed what your body can make. Arginine plays a pivotal role in collagen synthesis, which is essential for wound repair. Collagen acts as the structural framework of the healing tissue, ensuring wounds close effectively and regain strength.

Moreover, arginine enhances the immune system. It serves as a precursor to nitric oxide, a molecule that improves blood flow and supports immune function. Improved circulation ensures that oxygen and nutrients reach the wound site, accelerating the healing process. It can be particularly beneficial for patients with chronic wounds or burns.

Glutamine: The Healer's Helper
Glutamine is another amino acid that becomes essential during recovery periods. It is the primary fuel source for rapidly dividing cells, including those of the immune system and intestinal lining. After surgery, the body's demand for glutamine surges as it works to repair tissues and fend off infections. The

Journal of Burn Care & Research saw that in burn patients, glutamine not only sped up wound healing but also shortened hospital stays.

One of glutamine's standout features is its ability to maintain gut integrity. A healthy gut is crucial during recovery because it prevents harmful bacteria from entering the bloodstream, reducing the risk of post-surgical infections.

The Synergy of Arginine and Glutamine

While both amino acids independently support healing, research suggests their combined use can be even more beneficial. Together, they create a powerful synergy: arginine boosts collagen synthesis and immune function, while glutamine provides energy and maintains gut health, both essential for a swift recovery.

A noteworthy example comes from a targeted nutrition therapy review from *General Surgery News*, which showed that combining arginine and glutamine led to faster wound closure and reduced infection rates in patients with diabetic foot ulcers. This highlights the complementary roles these amino acids play in recovery.

How to Incorporate These Amino Acids

For patients undergoing surgery, incorporating arginine and glutamine can be achieved through a balanced diet rich in high-protein foods such as poultry, fish, dairy, and legumes. However, during intense recovery periods, supplementation may be beneficial, especially in cases where nutritional needs are heightened.

Collagen: Your Body's Building Block for Healing

Collagen is popularly known as a beauty supplement for how it promotes youthful skin. What most don't know is that it's the most abundant protein in your body, acting as the main structural protein found in skin, bones, muscles, tendons, and other connective tissues. Think of collagen as the "scaffolding" of the temple that provides strength and structure to your tissues. When you get an injury or have surgery, your body needs collagen to repair and rebuild damaged tissues. Research supports the wonderful effects of adding this to your nutrition plan. In burn patients, studies show that collagen supplementation can speed healing by up to 3.7 times and potentially reduce your stay at the hospital. Sports medicine research has found benefits for soft tissue injuries, with studies showing faster recovery from exercise-induced muscle damage.

You can support your body's natural collagen production through proper nutrition, particularly adequate protein intake and vitamin C, which is essential for collagen synthesis. While your body produces collagen naturally, research indicates that supplementation may be beneficial during periods of healing and recovery, particularly in cases of major surgery, burns, or significant tissue injury. While you are looking into supplement options, take note that studies have shown that hydrolyzed collagen supplements are better absorbed than non-hydrolyzed forms, with benefits observed at doses ranging from 10 to 15 grams daily.

Research-Supported Benefits of Collagen for Recovery

- Enhanced wound healing rates in surgical patients
- Improved recovery from burn injuries
- Better muscle repair after injury
- Reduced inflammation in joint injuries
- Potentially shortened hospital stays
- Improved skin healing and reduced scarring
- Enhanced soft tissue repair

While protein is crucial, other nutrients also play vital roles in recovery. We went over the following information in Chapter 2, however, here is a refresher keeping in mind all we just learned about amino acids:

- **Vitamin C:** Essential for collagen production and wound healing. Also acts as an antioxidant.
  - → Intake: 65–90 mg/day (up to 2000 mg/day safe).
  - → Sources: Citrus fruits, bell peppers, strawberries, broccoli.

- **Vitamin D:** Supports immune function and bone health.
  - → Intake: 600–800 IU/day (often recommended at 1000–2000 IU/day).
  - → Sources: Fatty fish, egg yolks, fortified foods, sunlight.

- **Vitamin A:** Crucial for cell growth and immune function
  - → Intake: 700–900 mcg (microgram) RAE (Retinol Activity Equivalents)/day.
  - → Sources: Sweet potatoes, carrots, spinach.

- **Zinc:** Vital for wound healing and immune support.
  - → Intake: 8–11 mg/day.
  - → Sources: Oysters, beef, pumpkin seeds, lentils.

- **Iron:** Supports oxygen transport, crucial if blood loss occurs.
  - → Intake: 8–18 mg/day.
  - → Sources: Red meat, poultry, fish, beans.

- **Magnesium**: Aids muscle and nerve function, may reduce inflammation.
  - → Intake: 310–420 mg/day.
  - → Sources: Nuts, seeds, whole grains, leafy greens.

PRACTICAL TIPS FOR INCREASING YOUR PROTEIN INTAKE

- Include a protein source with every meal and snack.
- Consider protein smoothies or shakes for an easy-to-consume protein boost.
- Greek yogurt is an excellent high-protein snack or breakfast option.
- Add beans or lentils to soups and salads for a plant-based protein boost.
- Keep hard-boiled eggs on hand for a quick, protein-rich snack.

Eating the Rainbow: Your Guide to Colorful Nutrition

COLOR GROUP	FOODS	KEY BENEFITS
Red Foods	Tomatoes	Rich in lycopene
	Red bell peppers	Packed with vitamin C
	Strawberries	Full of antioxidants
	Red apples	Good source of fiber
	Watermelon	Hydrating and nutrient-rich
	Cherries	Natural anti-inflammatory properties
Orange/ Yellow Foods	Carrots	Excellent for vitamin A and eye health
	Sweet potatoes	Rich in beta-carotene
	Orange bell peppers	High in vitamin C
	Mangoes	Good source of vitamins A and C
	Pineapple	Contains digestive enzymes
	Squash	Packed with nutrients and fiber

Green Foods	Spinach	Iron and vitamin K
	Broccoli	Rich in vitamins C and K
	Kale	Packed with antioxidants
	Avocados	Healthy fats and fiber
	Green beans	Good source of vitamins
	Cucumber	Hydrating and low-calorie
Purple/ Blue Foods	Blueberries	High in antioxidants
	Purple cabbage	Rich in protective compounds
	Eggplant	Good source of fiber
	Blackberries	Packed with vitamins
	Purple grapes	Contain resveratrol
	Plums	Rich in minerals
White/ Brown Foods	Mushrooms	Good source of vitamin D
	Cauliflower	Rich in fiber and vitamins
	Garlic	Natural immune booster
	Onions	Rich in antioxidants
	Potatoes	Good source of potassium
	White beans	Protein and fiber rich

QUICK COLORFUL EATING TIPS

- Try to include at least three different colors in each meal
- Eat fruits and vegetables both raw and cooked
- Choose seasonal options for best flavor and value
- Keep pre-cut options ready for easy snacking
- Mix colors in salads, stir-fries, and smoothies

Carbohydrate Loading: Fueling Your Body for Surgery

Imagine heading into surgery feeling a little stronger, a little less anxious, and knowing you've given your body a head start on healing. This is the idea behind carbohydrate loading—a simple yet powerful strategy that can make a significant difference in your surgical recovery.

Why Carbohydrate Loading Matters

1. **Tackling Insulin Resistance:** Surgery puts your body under stress, triggering insulin resistance—a condition where your cells don't use insulin effectively, leading to poor blood sugar control. This can slow down recovery and increase complications. Carbohydrate loading helps combat this by providing your body with a steady source of glucose, which reduces the stress-induced insulin resistance.
2. **Boosting Energy and Comfort:** Traditional fasting before surgery often leaves patients feeling weak, hungry, and anxious. Carbohydrate loading replaces fasting with a more comfortable option—clear carbohydrate-rich drinks up to two hours before surgery (if allowed by your surgeon). This not only improves energy levels but also reduces anxiety and discomfort.

3. **Shortened Hospital Stay and Faster Recovery**: Carbohydrate loading doesn't just make you feel better before surgery—it also helps you bounce back faster afterward. By maintaining your energy reserves, it supports quicker healing and a shorter hospital stay.
4. **Preserving Muscle Mass:** Surgery can take a toll on your body, including your muscles. Carbohydrate loading helps protect your muscle mass by preserving glycogen stores, the body's energy reserve, which can be depleted during surgery and recovery.

Fast vs. Slow Carbs

When we talk about carbohydrate loading, it's important to know the difference between fast carbs and slow carbs.

- **Fast Carbs:** These are simple sugars found in drinks like clear apple juice or sports drinks. They provide quick energy and are easy to digest—perfect for pre-surgery.
- **Slow Carbs:** Found in foods like whole grains, legumes, and vegetables, these take longer to break down and provide a steady energy release. While not suitable for the immediate pre-surgery window, they are excellent in the days leading up to surgery to maintain steady energy levels.

Home Hacks for Carbohydrate Loading

Two Days Before Surgery:

Focus on meals rich in slow carbs. Think whole grain pasta, brown rice, lentils, and sweet potatoes. These will build up your energy reserves gradually.

The Evening Before Surgery:

Enjoy a balanced dinner with a good mix of slow carbs, lean protein, and vegetables. A bowl of quinoa with grilled chicken and steamed broccoli is a great option.

Morning of Surgery (If Allowed)
Up to two hours before surgery, sip on clear carbohydrate drinks like diluted fruit juice (apple or grape) or a commercial carbohydrate drink specifically designed for surgery prep. This provides quick, digestible energy to fuel your body without overloading the digestive system.

DIY Carbohydrate Drink
Mix 200 ml of clear apple juice with 200 ml of water and a pinch of salt. This simple drink can help maintain energy levels and hydration before surgery.

By understanding and incorporating carbohydrate loading into your surgical prep, you're giving your body the tools it needs to handle surgery with resilience and recover more efficiently. Always consult with your healthcare provider to tailor this approach to your specific needs.

Foods to Avoid Before Surgery

High-fat and fried foods
These can slow digestion and increase the risk of aspiration during anesthesia. They may also contribute to postoperative nausea.

- Examples: Fried chicken, French fries, fatty cuts of meat, creamy sauces, and pastries.
- Timeframe: Avoid for at least 24 hours before surgery.

Foods that increase bleeding risk
Some foods and supplements can thin the blood, potentially increasing the risk of excessive bleeding during surgery.

- Examples: Garlic, ginger, ginseng, and high doses of fish oil supplements.
- Timeframe: Discontinue use at least 7–10 days before surgery, or as directed by your surgeon.

Alcohol

Alcohol can interact with anesthesia and pain medications, and may increase the risk of bleeding and other complications.

- Recommendation: Avoid alcohol for at least 48 hours before surgery. Ideally, abstain for a week or more prior to your procedure.

Caffeine

While small amounts of caffeine are generally not problematic, excessive caffeine intake can lead to dehydration and increased heart rate, which can be risky during surgery.

- Recommendation: Limit caffeine to one cup of coffee or tea per day in the days leading up to surgery. Some doctors may advise complete avoidance 24–48 hours before the procedure.

Herbal supplements and teas

Many herbal products can interact with anesthesia or affect blood clotting.

- Examples: St. John's Wort, Echinacea, Valerian root, Kava kava.
- Timeframe: Generally, discontinue all herbal supplements 2–3 weeks before surgery, but always consult with your healthcare provider for specific guidance.

Practical tips for avoiding problematic foods:

1. Inform your surgeon about all medications, supplements, and herbal products you're taking. Especially if you regularly use blood thinners such as Aspirin, Advil, and Excedrin.
2. When in doubt about a food or supplement, ask your healthcare provider.
3. Focus on simple, easily digestible foods in the days leading up to surgery.
4. Keep a food diary in the week before surgery to ensure you're avoiding potentially problematic foods.

Hydration

You may already know how important staying hydrated is for daily life and health. The same goes for surgery, but perhaps even more so. Proper hydration is crucial for optimal surgical outcomes. It supports circulation, aids digestion, and helps regulate body temperature. Adequate hydration can also help prevent complications such as constipation and urinary tract infections, which are common after surgery.

Benefits of proper hydration include:

- Improved circulation: Adequate hydration ensures that your blood is not too thick, which stabilizes blood pressure during surgery and helps deliver nutrients to tissues effectively.
- Support for digestive health: Hydration helps prevent constipation, a common side effect of pain medications and reduced mobility after surgery.
- Temperature regulation: Hydration helps your body maintain its temperature, which is important during surgery when your body is exposed to different environmental factors.
- Reduced risk of complications: Good hydration can help reduce the risk of blood clots and support kidney function.

HYDRATION STATUS CHECK

URINE COLOR	MEANING	ACTION NEEDED
Clear	Over-hydrated	Reduce intake
Pale yellow	Optimal	Maintain current intake
Dark yellow	Dehydrated	Increase water intake
Amber	Severely dehydrated	Seek medical attention

Hydration Recommendations

- Aim for 8–10 glasses (64–80 ounces) of water a day, unless otherwise directed by your healthcare provider.
- In some cases, electrolyte drinks may be recommended to ensure balanced hydration, especially if you're at risk of electrolyte imbalances.
- Follow your doctor's instructions on when to stop drinking before surgery. Generally, clear liquids are allowed up to 2 hours before the procedure, but this can vary based on the type of surgery and individual factors.

PRACTICAL TIPS FOR STAYING HYDRATED

- Carry a reusable water bottle with you and refill it throughout the day.
- Set reminders on your phone to drink water regularly.
- Consume water-rich foods like fruits and vegetables to supplement your fluid intake.
- Herbal teas (without caffeine) can count towards your daily fluid intake.
- Monitor your urine color—pale yellow indicates good hydration.

Remember, these guidelines are general, and it's crucial to follow the specific instructions provided by your surgical team. They will take into account your individual health status and the nature of your surgery when providing nutritional and hydration guidance.

By focusing on these key areas—building a strong nutritional foundation, consuming essential nutrients, implementing carbohydrate loading when appropriate, avoiding problematic foods, and maintaining proper hydration—you can significantly improve your body's ability to withstand the stress of surgery and recover more effectively. Always work closely with your healthcare team to create a personalized plan that best suits your individual needs and the specific requirements of your upcoming surgery.

5

Recovering with Mindfulness & Meditation

Why Meditation?

Throughout this book, we've explored the profound impact that nutrition has on the body's healing processes. But healing is multidimensional, involving not just the physical body but also the mind. This is where meditation enters the picture—as a powerful complementary practice that can significantly enhance recovery and overall wellbeing.

Meditation, at its core, is a set of techniques designed to enhance awareness, cultivate attention, and achieve mental clarity. While often associated with spiritual traditions, meditation has evolved into a secular practice backed by a growing body of scientific research documenting its benefits for both physical and mental health.

My Personal Journey with Meditation

My own relationship with meditation began long before my heart surgery, but it was during my recovery that I truly came to appreciate its profound healing potential. In the weeks leading up to my procedure, I experienced the anxiety that inevitably accompanies such a significant health challenge. Despite my medical knowledge and understanding of the surgical process, I found myself wrestling with worry and uncertainty.

Meditation became my anchor during this turbulent time. Through regular practice, I was able to quiet the endless stream of "what-ifs" and stay grounded in the present moment. I developed a series of guided meditations specifically designed to address pre-surgical anxiety, promote healing, and cultivate gratitude throughout the recovery process. These practices were so beneficial to my own healing journey that I've since made them available through my app to help others navigate similar challenges.

After surgery, meditation helped me manage pain with less reliance on medication. It allowed me to tune into my body's signals without becoming overwhelmed by discomfort. Most importantly, it gave me a tool to maintain a positive outlook despite the inevitable ups and downs of recovery.

What struck me most was how meditation helped me transform my perspective on the entire experience. Rather than viewing surgery as simply something to "get through," meditation helped me approach it as an opportunity for growth and deeper self-understanding. This shift in mindset didn't just make recovery more bearable—it made it meaningful.

The Science Behind Meditation and Surgical Recovery

While personal experiences like mine are compelling, the scientific evidence supporting meditation's benefits for surgical patients is equally impressive. Research has shown that regular meditation practice can positively impact numerous aspects of the surgical journey.

Studies have consistently shown that meditation can help reduce preoperative anxiety, a common challenge for surgical patients. Research done in 2010 for an oncology study found that patients using guided imagery prior to surgery reported significantly lower anxiety levels. Similarly, a randomized controlled trial in 2006 demonstrated reduced anxiety both pre-surgery and during treatment for women with cancer who practiced mindfulness-based art therapy.

This reduction in anxiety is more than just a matter of comfort—lower anxiety levels are associated with better surgical outcomes and fewer complications.

Pain Management

One of the most well-documented benefits of meditation is pain reduction. A groundbreaking 2011 study published in *The Journal of Neuroscience* found that mindfulness meditation reduced pain intensity by 40 percent and unpleasantness by 57 percent. Brain imaging showed activation in brain areas that reduce pain perception, providing a neurological explanation for these effects.

Additionally, research published in the *Journal of the American Medical Association* (*JAMA*) in 2016 demonstrated that mindfulness improved pain and function in chronic pain sufferers. For you, this might look like not having to rely as much on pain medication, which carries its own risks and side effects.

Immune Function

It may seem far-fetched to learn meditation can help your immune system. But like I mentioned at the beginning of this book, your body is capable of astounding things. Further, your mind and emotions have a profound impact on how you feel physically. Research has demonstrated that meditation practices can positively influence immune function—a critical factor in wound healing and infection prevention. A landmark study published in *Psychosomatic Medicine* in 2003 found increased antibody production following influenza vaccinations in meditation practitioners, suggesting an enhanced immune response.

A systematic review (a process of summarizing and analyzing all available research on a topic) published in the *Annals of the New York Academy of Sciences* in 2016 examined randomized controlled trials and found evidence that mindfulness enhances immune markers and affects gene expression, potentially supporting better healing outcomes.

Inflammatory Response

If you meditate, you even have the power to regulate your body's inflammatory response. Impressive, right? A comprehensive review published in *Frontiers in Immunology* found that meditation and similar practices downregulated pro-inflammatory genes.

Further supporting this, research featured in *Brain, Behavior, and Immunity* showed that mindfulness-based stress reduction reduced pro-inflammatory gene expression, potentially creating a more favorable internal environment for healing.

Sleep Quality

Many surgical patients struggle with sleep disruption, which can impede your healing. Research published in *JAMA Internal Medicine* showed that mindfulness meditation significantly improved sleep quality and reduced daytime impairment among older adults with sleep disturbances. Better sleep supports the body's natural healing mechanisms and can accelerate recovery.

Types of Meditation for Surgical Recovery

There are many approaches to meditation, each with unique characteristics and potential benefits. Three forms that have shown particular promise for surgical patients include:

Mindfulness Meditation

This practice involves paying attention to the present moment with an attitude of openness and non-judgment. To try this out, you can access various tools for free online. I have also created an app called Mendora (scan QR code below to access the app) which gives you access not only to various meditations but numerous healing recipes and tips. If you still think meditation is only for hippies, remember there is neurological evidence that shows mindfulness can literally change your brain's response to pain. So, if there is a chance you can make your surgical journal more comfortable, wouldn't it be worth the effort?

As a surgical patient, mindfulness can help you manage pain by changing how your brain perceives and responds to physical sensations. It also helps create space between thoughts and emotions, allowing you to experience anxiety or discomfort without becoming overwhelmed by these feelings.

To access recovery meditations, scan the QR code above.

Mantra-Based Meditation (Transcendental Meditation)

Practices like transcendental meditation (TM) involve silently repeating a mantra (a word or sound) to facilitate a state of relaxed awareness. A study published in *Circulation: Cardiovascular Quality and Outcomes* found that TM reduced the risk of death, myocardial infarction, and stroke by an impressive 48 percent in patients with coronary heart disease.

The American Heart Association, specifically recommended TM as an approach for lowering blood pressure—an important consideration for many surgical patients, particularly those undergoing cardiac procedures.

Guided Imagery Meditation (Positive Visualization Technique)

Guided imagery is a mind-body practice in which a listener is led through a calming visualization, typically lasting 5 to 10 minutes. This technique begins with deep relaxation and continues with positive suggestions and vivid mental imagery focused on healing and recovery.

For surgical patients, guided imagery may involve visualizing a smooth and successful surgery, tissues regenerating and healing optimally, a reduction in pain or inflammation, and a return to normal function and daily activities. This method harnesses the power of the mind-body connection, where mental imagery can influence physiological responses.

Scientific evidence supports its use: research published in the *American Journal of Critical Care* and other peer-reviewed journals has shown that guided imagery can significantly reduce post-operative pain and anxiety while enhancing overall recovery quality—particularly in patients undergoing coronary artery bypass grafting and other major surgeries.

Integrating Meditation into Your Surgical Journey

As you can tell, mindfulness has the potential to drastically improve your healing journey. If you're preparing for surgery, consider incorporating meditation into your preparation and recovery plan. Here are some practical suggestions:

Start small
Even five to ten minutes of daily meditation can produce benefits. You can gradually increase the duration as you become more comfortable with the practice. **Consistency matters**: Regular practice, even if brief, tends to yield better results than occasional longer sessions.

Find what works for you
Explore different meditation styles to discover what resonates with your preferences and needs.

Use available resources
Guided meditations specifically designed for surgical patients can be particularly helpful, especially if you're new to meditation. The Mendora app is an excellent start. We have curated multiple guided meditations to help you with anxiety, sleep, recovery and healing.

Continue post-surgery
While you may need to adapt your practice during the immediate recovery period, maintaining meditation throughout recovery can support ongoing healing.

Meditation for Everyday Life

While our focus in this chapter has been on meditation's benefits for surgical recovery, it's worth noting that these practices offer advantages that extend far beyond the medical context. Regular meditation has been associated with reduced stress, improved emotional regulation, enhanced attention, and better overall quality of life.

Many patients who begin meditating in preparation for surgery find that they want to continue the practice indefinitely. You might also discover that the same mental clarity and emotional balance that helped you through surgery serves you well in navigating life's everyday challenges.

In my own life, meditation has become as essential to my wellbeing as proper nutrition and physical activity. The mental resilience and emotional equilibrium it fosters have proven invaluable not just in times of health challenges, but in all aspects of my personal and professional life.

TAKEAWAY

As we close this chapter, I invite you to consider meditation not just as an adjunct to your surgical recovery, but as a valuable life skill that can enhance your overall well being. The mind and body are inextricably connected—by nurturing both, you create the optimal conditions for healing and health.

Whether you're facing surgery or simply seeking to improve your quality of life, meditation offers a time-tested approach to cultivating inner calm, managing physical discomfort, and fostering a positive outlook. When combined with the nutritional strategies we've explored in previous chapters, meditation creates a powerful foundation for healing, recovery, and lasting wellness.

Remember, healing is a holistic process that encompasses body, mind, and spirit. By honoring all of these dimensions, you give yourself the greatest opportunity to not just recover, but to thrive.

6

Pre-Surgery Checklist

In order to ease anxiety and make your life easier, I have created a list to have on hand that will set you up for success before surgery. I aimed to combine all that we have discussed so far into this list, including actionable steps. Do this well in advance, so that all you need to worry about later is resting and healing. That alone will take enough of your energy and focus, so a bit of forethought will have you thanking yourself later. Without further ado, let's dive into this chapter which provides a comprehensive checklist to help you prepare in the weeks leading up to your procedure. These are just general guidelines and you should always check with your physician about their specific recommendations for the type of surgery you are having.

Nutritional Preparation (2–4 Weeks Before Surgery)

- ☐ **IMPLEMENT A HIGH-PROTEIN DIET:**
  - → Aim for 1.2-2.0 g of protein per kg of body weight daily.
  - → Include lean meats, fish, eggs, dairy, and plant-based proteins in your meals.
  - → Consider protein supplements if recommended by your healthcare provider.

- ☐ **BEGIN RECOMMENDED SUPPLEMENTS:**
  - → Multivitamin: Ensure you're meeting basic nutritional needs.
  - → Vitamin C: 500–1000 mg daily to support collagen production and wound healing.
  - → Vitamin D: 1000–2000 IU daily, especially if deficient.
  - → Discuss any additional supplements with your doctor.

- ☐ **START HYDRATION REGIMEN:**
  - → Aim for 8–10 glasses of water daily.
  - → Monitor urine color (pale yellow indicates good hydration).
  - → Reduce caffeine and alcohol intake.

Meal Planning and Prep

- ☐ **GROCERY SHOPPING GUIDE:**
  - → Stock up on easily digestible, nutrient-rich foods.
  - → Choose foods high in protein, fiber, and essential vitamins.
  - → Avoid processed and high-fat foods.

- ☐ **MEAL PREP STRATEGIES:**
  - → Prepare and freeze portion-sized meals for easy post-surgery nutrition.
  - → Make nutrient-dense smoothies and freeze in individual portions.
  - → Cook large batches of soups and stews rich in vegetables and lean proteins.

Lifestyle Adjustments

- ☐ **EXERCISE RECOMMENDATIONS:**
  - → Engage in regular moderate exercise to improve overall health.
  - → Focus on strength training to build muscle mass before surgery.
  - → Practice deep breathing exercises to improve lung function.

- ☐ **STRESS REDUCTION TECHNIQUES:**
  - → Start a daily meditation practice (5–10 minutes daily).
  - → Try progressive muscle relaxation techniques.
  - → Consider yoga or tai chi for mind-body balance.

Medical and Logistical Preparation

- [ ] **MEDICATION REVIEW:**
  - → Discuss all current medications with your surgeon.
  - → Prepare a list of allergies and previous surgical experiences.
  - → Stop blood-thinning medications as advised by your doctor.

- [ ] **HOME PREPARATION:**
  - → Arrange for post-surgery care and transportation.
  - → Prepare a comfortable recovery area in your home.
  - → Gather loose, comfortable clothing for after the surgery.

- [ ] **COMMUNICATION:**
  - → Inform family and friends about your surgery date.
  - → Arrange for time off work and delegate responsibilities.
  - → Discuss expected recovery time and limitations with your surgeon.

7

Day-of-Surgery Checklist

We have learned all about vitamins, minerals, and the key components for making sure your nutrition is the best it can be for an optimal healing process. You have eaten well, prepared your home space, and done everything you can to get ready for this day, and now it has arrived. While this is exciting, I'm sure it can also make you slightly nervous. Being well-prepared the day of your surgery can help reduce stress and ensure everything goes smoothly. To that end, this chapter provides a comprehensive checklist for the night before and the morning of your surgery.

Night Before Surgery

- ☐ **FINAL MEAL GUIDELINES:**
  - → Have a light, easily digestible dinner.
  - → Avoid fatty, spicy, or heavy foods.
  - → Follow any specific dietary instructions from your surgeon.

- ☐ **HYDRATION INSTRUCTIONS:**
  - → Continue to hydrate well throughout the evening.
  - → Stop drinking fluids at the time specified by your healthcare provider (usually midnight).

- ☐ **PERSONAL HYGIENE:**
  - → Take a shower or bath using antibacterial soap if instructed.
  - → Do not apply lotions, perfumes, or deodorants after bathing.
  - → Remove nail polish and do not wear makeup

- ☐ **PREPARATION FOR THE MORNING:**
  - → Lay out comfortable, loose-fitting clothes for the next day.
  - → Prepare a small bag with essentials (ID, insurance card, list of medications).
  - → Set multiple alarms to ensure you wake up on time.

Morning of Surgery

- ☐ **FASTING COMPLIANCE:**
  - → Do not eat or drink anything unless specifically instructed by your doctor.
  - → If allowed clear liquids, stop intake 2 hours before scheduled surgery time.

- ☐ **MEDICATION MANAGEMENT:**
  - → Take only the medications approved by your anesthesiologist with a small sip of water.
  - → Bring a list of all your regular medications and their dosages.

- ☐ **CARBOHYDRATE LOADING (IF RECOMMENDED):**
  - → If advised, consume the prescribed amount of carbohydrate drink 2–3 hours before surgery.
  - → Follow exact instructions provided by your healthcare team.

- ☐ **FINAL PREPARATIONS:**
  - → Wear comfortable, loose-fitting clothes.
  - → Do not wear contact lenses, jewelry, or body piercings.
  - → Bring any medical devices you regularly use (e.g., CPAP machine, insulin pump).

- ☐ **ARRIVAL AT THE HOSPITAL OR SURGERY CENTER:**
  - → Arrive at the specified time (usually 2 hours before scheduled surgery).
  - → Bring a form of identification and your insurance information.
  - → Have a family member or friend accompany you.

8

Post-Surgery Recovery Checklist

You made it. By this point, your surgery is complete and everything hopefully went smoothly. Congratulations! Now that you have created a strong foundation of nutrition leading up to surgery, all that you have to do now is maintain it. Your healing journey officially begins. How you treat your body over the days and weeks immediately following your surgery has a big impact on your recovery. Ideally you have also enlisted your family members or roommates as accomplices for this crucial chapter when support is most welcome. As you will see, this chapter provides a comprehensive checklist to guide you through the initial recovery phase and beyond. Recovery is a journey, and every person's path is unique. Use this checklist as a guide but always follow the specific instructions provided by your healthcare team.

Immediate Post-Op Period (0-48 hours)

- ☐ **HYDRATION TRACKING:**
  - → Sip water or clear fluids as allowed by your care team.
  - → Monitor urine output and color.
  - → Report any difficulties with urination to your nurse.

- ☐ **INTRODUCING CLEAR LIQUIDS AND SOFT FOODS:**
  - → Start with ice chips or small sips of water when allowed.
  - → Gradually introduce clear broths and gelatin as tolerated.
  - → Progress to soft foods as per your doctor's instructions.

- ☐ **PAIN MANAGEMENT:**
  - → Use the pain scale to communicate your comfort level.
  - → Take pain medication as prescribed.
  - → Report any uncontrolled pain or adverse reactions to medications.

- ☐ **EARLY MOBILIZATION:**
  - → Follow instructions for getting out of bed safely.
  - → Perform any prescribed in-bed exercises.
  - → Take short walks with assistance as recommended by your care team.

Early Recovery (Days 3-7)

- [ ] **GRADUALLY INCREASING PROTEIN INTAKE:**
  - → Aim to meet the recommended protein intake (1.2-2.0 g/kg/day).
  - → Include protein sources in every meal and snack.
  - → Consider protein supplements if recommended by your dietitian.

- [ ] **REINTRODUCING SOLID FOODS:**
  - → Follow your doctor's guidance on diet progression.
  - → Introduce new foods one at a time to monitor tolerance.
  - → Focus on nutrient-dense, easily digestible options.

- [ ] **SYMPTOM TRACKING:**
  - → Keep a daily log of pain levels, medication usage, and any side effects.
  - → Monitor the surgical site for signs of infection (redness, swelling, discharge).
  - → Track your bowel movements and report any constipation or diarrhea.

- [ ] **PHYSICAL ACTIVITY:**
  - → Gradually increase your activity level as advised by your care team.
  - → Continue with prescribed exercises or physical therapy.
  - → Listen to your body and rest when needed.

Ongoing Recovery (Week 2 and Onward)

- ☐ **MEETING DAILY NUTRITIONAL GOALS:**
  - → Continue to focus on high-protein, nutrient-dense foods.
  - → Incorporate a variety of fruits and vegetables for micronutrients.
  - → Stay hydrated with water and clear fluids.

- ☐ **MEDICATION MANAGEMENT:**
  - → Follow your prescribed medication schedule.
  - → Discuss any side effects or concerns with your healthcare provider.
  - → Do not stop any medications without consulting your doctor.

- ☐ **WOUND CARE:**
  - → Follow specific instructions for caring for your surgical site.
  - → Attend follow-up appointments for wound checks.
  - → Report any signs of infection promptly.

- ☐ **GRADUAL RETURN TO NORMAL ACTIVITIES:**
  - → Follow your surgeon's guidelines for returning to work and daily activities.
  - → Gradually increase physical activity as allowed.
  - → Avoid heavy lifting or strenuous exercise until cleared by your doctor.

9

Conquering Post-Surgery Challenges Through Your Diet

Recovering from surgery isn't always the smooth, linear process we hope it will be. Sure, we all imagine a steady climb toward feeling better, but the truth is often more complicated. Along the way, you might find yourself dealing with constipation, a lack of appetite, overwhelming fatigue, or even a dip in your immune defenses. These challenges are common, but they can feel like roadblocks to recovery.

Here's the good news: what you eat—and how you eat—can make a world of difference. Your diet has the power to support your healing, ease discomfort, and give your body the tools it needs to rebuild. This chapter is designed to be your guide, offering practical, easy-to-follow strategies to tackle the most common post-surgery hurdles.

Let's walk through it together.

Dealing with Constipation

If you've been feeling backed up after surgery, you're not alone. Constipation is one of the most frequent post-op complaints. Pain medications (especially opioids), reduced activity, and changes in your eating habits all contribute to slower digestion.

Why Constipation Happens

Opioids slow down your gut's natural rhythm, while decreased movement and low fiber intake make matters worse. It's frustrating, uncomfortable, and can make recovery feel even harder. But the solution starts with what's on your plate (and in your glass).

Add Fiber Gradually
Fiber is your digestive system's best friend. It helps move things along by bulking up your stool and making it easier to pass. There are two types of fiber, and both are helpful:

- **Soluble Fiber:** Found in oats, apples, and carrots, this type softens stool. Prunes, which are high in soluble fiber and sorbitol, are particularly effective in alleviating constipation.
- **Insoluble Fiber:** Found in whole grains, leafy greens, and nuts, this type helps stool move through your intestines more efficiently.

Practical Steps

- Start your morning with oatmeal topped with berries and a sprinkle of flaxseeds.
- Include a serving of vegetables with every meal—think roasted broccoli at lunch or a spinach side salad at dinner.
- Snack on prunes (yes, they work!) or a small handful of almonds.

Don't Forget Hydration

Here's the catch: fiber only works if you're drinking enough water. Without it, fiber can actually make constipation worse. Proper hydration softens stools and works synergistically with fiber to improve gut motility.

Practical Tips

- Sip water throughout the day instead of chugging large amounts at once.
- Include broth-based soups, which hydrate while offering nutrients.
- Avoid sugary drinks and caffeine, which can dehydrate you.

Move a Little

Even light activity, like a short walk around your house or gentle stretching, can wake up your digestive system and help relieve constipation.

Managing Appetite Loss

After surgery, you might feel like food is the last thing on your mind. Appetite loss is normal—it's often triggered by anesthesia, pain medications, and the stress your body is under. However, this lack of appetite can be partly due to changes in your body's hormonal and immune responses to surgery.

Small Steps, Big Impact

Eating smaller, more frequent meals is often easier than trying to tackle a big plate of food. Think of it as grazing throughout the day rather than sitting down for three large meals.

Practical Examples

- A boiled egg with a slice of avocado.
- A smoothie made with banana, Greek yogurt, and protein powder.
- A handful of nuts and dried fruit.

Choose Nutrient-Dense Foods

When your appetite is low, make every bite count. Focus on foods that pack a lot of nutrition into smaller portions.

Practical Examples

- **Avocados:** Full of healthy fats and calories.
- **Greek Yogurt:** Rich in protein and probiotics.
- **Nuts and Seeds:** Calorie-dense and packed with vitamins and minerals.

Appeal to Your Senses

Sometimes it's not about hunger but how the food looks and smells. A colorful plate with fresh ingredients can make eating more appealing.

Practical Ideas

- Add vibrant fruits like berries or citrus to your meals.
- Sprinkle fresh herbs or lemon zest for an aromatic boost.

If solid foods still feel like too much, try liquid options like bone broths, soups, or smoothies. They're easier to consume but still deliver nutrients.

Combating Fatigue

Fatigue can feel overwhelming after surgery, but it's your body's way of saying it needs extra energy to heal. While rest is crucial, so is eating foods that provide steady, lasting energy.

Energy-Boosting Foods

- **Iron-Rich Foods:** Iron helps carry oxygen to your cells, and low levels can leave you feeling drained.
  → Examples: Red meat, spinach, lentils, and fortified cereals.
  → Tip: Pair iron-rich foods with vitamin C (like spinach with a squeeze of lemon) to boost absorption.
- **B Vitamins:** These are essential for converting food into energy.
  → Sources: Eggs, whole grains, and leafy greens.
- **Complex Carbohydrates:** These provide steady energy without blood sugar crashes.
  → Sources: Quinoa, oats, and sweet potatoes.

Practical Steps

- Add a serving of lentils to your lunch or dinner.
- Start your day with a whole grain toast topped with avocado and an egg.
- Snack on a small handful of walnuts or almonds.

Supporting Immune Function

Your immune system works overtime after surgery to prevent infections and help your wounds heal. Giving it the right nutrients can make its job easier.

Immune-Boosting Foods

- **Vitamin C:** Known for its role in boosting immunity, it also promotes collagen production for wound healing.
  → Sources: Oranges, strawberries, bell peppers, and broccoli.
- **Zinc:** Helps with wound healing and supports immune cells.
  → Sources: Shellfish, pumpkin seeds, and chickpeas.
- **Probiotics:** A healthy gut is closely linked to a strong immune system.
  → Sources: Yogurt with live cultures, kefir, and fermented vegetables.

Garlic's Hidden Power

Garlic contains allicin, a compound with natural antibacterial and antiviral properties. Add fresh garlic to soups or roasted vegetables for an extra immune boost.

Supplements to Consider

- Multivitamins: They cover nutritional gaps if your diet is limited
- Vitamin D: Especially important if you're spending a lot of time indoors.
- Probiotics: They support gut health when fermented foods aren't an option.

TAKEAWAY

YOUR PATH TO RECOVERY

Surgery recovery is a journey, not a sprint. It's normal to face challenges along the way, but with the right strategies, you can tackle them head-on. Whether it's drinking more water to ease constipation, eating a handful of nuts to combat fatigue, or adding colorful ingredients to make meals more appealing, every small step adds up.

You've got this. Take it one day—and one bite—at a time.

10

Long-Term Nutrition to Thrive

As I sit in my office reviewing post-operative photos with a patient of mine named Sarah, a professional violinist who underwent orbital surgery six months ago at the time of this writing, she shares an observation that deeply resonates with me. "Dr. Parsa," she says, touching the barely visible scar near her eye, "this experience has completely changed how I think about food. It's not just about healing anymore—it's about nourishing my whole body."

Her words take me back to my own journey with my finger injury, which we discussed in the Prologue. What began as a desperate search for alternatives to surgery evolved into a profound understanding of nutrition's role in our body's incredible capacity for healing. Now, years later, many of the dietary changes I made during that healing period have become permanent fixtures in my life—not because I'm still healing, but because I've witnessed firsthand how proper nutrition can enhance my body's natural resilience.

This chapter marks a momentous transition in your healing journey. We're moving beyond the immediate post-surgery phase to explore how the nutritional principles we've discussed can support your long-term health and vitality. Remember those evolutionary connections we explored in Chapter 2—how our bodies have developed over millions of years in concert with the natural world? And recall our discussion in Chapter 3 about the challenges posed by modern food systems? Now, we'll bridge these concepts to create a sustainable approach to nutrition that honors both our evolutionary heritage and the realities of contemporary life.

The Transition: From Healing to Thriving

Let me share another story that illustrates this transition perfectly. Michael, a fifty-two-year-old executive who underwent extensive facial surgery, came to me frustrated about six weeks after his surgery. "The initial healing is going well," he said, "but I feel stuck. I'm afraid to deviate from my post-surgery diet, yet I know I need to move forward."

Michael's concern is common and understandable. The transition from a focused healing diet to a long-term nutritional strategy can feel daunting. Let's break this down into manageable steps, building on what we've learned about our body's nutritional needs.

Step 1: Honoring Your Body's Wisdom

Remember our discussion about the "sacred dance of life and nutrients" from Chapter 2 This same dance continues long after your initial healing. Your body carries within it the wisdom of billions of years of evolution, and learning to listen to its signals is crucial for this transition.

Practical Application

- Start with a food journal, noting not just what you eat but how different foods make you feel.
- Pay attention to your energy levels, digestion, and overall vitality.
- Watch for signs of inflammation or sensitivity.

Step 2: Reintroducing Foods Mindfully

Just as we discussed how our ancient ancestors adapted their diets based on their environment, you'll need to adapt your diet thoughtfully during this transition. This isn't about rushing back to your pre-surgery eating habits—it's about consciously creating a new, more nourishing approach to food.

The Traffic Light System for Food Reintroduction

Green Light Foods (Start Here):

- Nutrient-dense whole foods that were part of your healing diet
- Foods rich in the essential macronutrients we explored in Chapter 2
- Easily digestible proteins and complex carbohydrates

Yellow Light Foods (Introduce Gradually):

- More complex dishes combining multiple ingredients
- Foods that might require more digestive effort
- New sources of protein or fiber

Red Light Foods (Approach with Caution):

- Processed foods containing additives we discussed in Chapter 3
- Known inflammatory triggers
- Foods that previously caused sensitivity

Building Your Forever Foundation

Last year, I treated Elena, a chef who lost her sense of taste temporarily after head trauma. During her recovery, she made an insightful observation: "Without being able to taste, I had to think about food differently—purely as nourishment for healing. Now that my taste is returning, I want to combine both perspectives: the joy of flavor and the power of nutrition."

Elena's experience perfectly illustrates the approach we want to take. Let's build on our understanding of macro and micronutrients from Chapter 2 to create a sustainable nutritional foundation.

The Evolutionary Blueprint

Remember how we discussed the intricate dance between nutrients and life that evolved over billions of years? Your long-term nutrition strategy should honor this ancient wisdom while adapting to modern realities.

1. The Protein Palette

Think of proteins as your body's continuing renovation crew. While the intense repair work of early healing may be complete, your body still needs quality protein for maintenance and renewal.

Strategic Sources

- Wild-caught fish (rich in both protein and anti-inflammatory omega-3s)
- Pasture-raised meats (higher in nutrients than their factory-farmed counterparts)
- Legumes and pulses (providing both protein and fiber)
- Seeds and nuts (offering protein plus healthy fats)

Implementation Tip

Aim for protein diversity. As one of my patients, Tom, a vegetarian athlete, discovered, rotating through different protein sources ensures a broader amino acid profile and helps prevent food sensitivities that can develop from overconsumption of any single source.

2. The Carbohydrate Conundrum

Here's where our modern food landscape poses particular challenges. As we discussed in Chapter 3, many contemporary carbohydrate sources bear little resemblance to their ancestral counterparts.

Optimal Choices

- Whole grains in their least processed forms
- Starchy vegetables like sweet potatoes and squash
- Fiber-rich fruits and vegetables
- Limited quantities of natural sweeteners

Quality Markers

- Minimal processing
- High fiber content
- Low glycemic impact
- Rich in complementary nutrients

3. The Fat Factor: Beyond Healing

Remember our discussion about the essential role of fats in cellular repair in chapter 2? Their importance doesn't diminish after initial healing.

Strategic Sources

- Cold-pressed oils (olive, avocado)
- Whole food fats (avocados, nuts, seeds)
- Omega-3 rich foods (fatty fish, chia seeds)
- Limited quantities of saturated fats from quality sources

Navigating the Modern Food Maze

One of my patients, David, a sixty-five-year-old grandfather, recently shared his strategy for grocery shopping: "I stick to the perimeter of the store where the real food is, and when I venture into the middle aisles, I remember your warnings about those European banned ingredients."

David's approach is smart. Let's build on our Chapter 3 discussion about food industry challenges to create a practical strategy for long-term nutrition.

The Clean Food Protocol:

1. *Primary Defense:*
   → Choose whole, unprocessed foods whenever possible
   → Verify sources (local, organic when feasible)
   → Read labels vigilantly (remember our discussion of banned additives)

2. *Strategic Shopping:*
    - → Prioritize fresh produce
    - → Choose pastured, wild, or organic animal products
    - → Look for minimal ingredient lists
    - → Avoid artificial additives and preservatives
3. *Kitchen Wisdom:*
    - → Cook from scratch when possible
    - → Use traditional food preparation methods
    - → Store food properly to maintain nutrient content
    - → Batch cook to make healthy eating convenient

The Supplement Question

I often think back to my finger injury and how targeted supplementation played a key role in my recovery. However, as I tell my patients, supplements in your long-term strategy should be just that—supplemental to a nutrient-dense diet.

Core Supplements to Consider

1. *Foundation Support:*
    - → High-quality multivitamin (to address potential gaps from modern food)
    - → Vitamin D3 (especially important for indoor lifestyles)
    - → Omega-3s (if not consuming adequate fatty fish)
2. *Situational Support:*
    - → Probiotics (particularly after antibiotics or if consuming primarily conventional foods)
    - → Magnesium (often depleted in modern soils)
    - → Specific nutrients based on your individual needs and lab work

Monitoring Your Progress

Remember Sarah, our violinist from the beginning of this chapter? She developed an elegant system for tracking her nutritional status, inspired by how she tunes her violin—regular, careful adjustments based on clear feedback. Below are some factors you can track in your own journal.

Key Indicators to Track

1. *Physical Markers:*
   - → Energy levels throughout the day
   - → Sleep quality
   - → Digestion and elimination
   - → Skin health
   - → Exercise recovery
2. *Regular Assessments:*
   - → Basic blood work (annually or as recommended)
   - → Vitamin D levels
   - → Iron status
   - → Inflammatory markers
3. *Subjective Measures:*
   - → Overall well-being
   - → Mental clarity
   - → Stress resilience
   - → Physical performance

TAKEAWAY

—

THE PATH FORWARD

As we conclude this chapter, I'm reminded of what Elena, our chef, said six months after her recovery: "This journey has given me a new recipe for life—one where every meal is an opportunity to nourish not just my body, but my future."

Your healing journey has equipped you with profound insights about your body's nutritional needs. Use this knowledge to create a sustainable approach to nutrition that honors both your body's ancient wisdom and your modern lifestyle.

KEY ACTIONS

- Transition gradually from healing to maintenance nutrition
- Focus on nutrient-dense, whole foods
- Navigate modern food challenges with informed choices
- Use supplements strategically
- Monitor and adjust your approach based on clear feedback

Remember, this isn't about perfection—it's about progress. Every meal is an opportunity to nourish your body and support its incredible capacity for renewal and vitality.

11

Easy Delicious & Nutritious Recipes

Throughout this book, we've explored the profound connection between nutrition and healing. We've delved into the science of how specific nutrients support your body's recovery processes, examined the challenges of modern food systems, and provided guidance for optimizing your diet before and after surgery. Now, it's time to put theory into practice with a collection of recipes designed to make healthy eating not just beneficial, but genuinely enjoyable.

One of the most persistent myths about nutritious eating is that it must be bland, boring, or restrictive. Nothing could be further from the truth. When we embrace whole, unprocessed foods in their natural state, we discover a world of vibrant flavors, satisfying textures, and endless culinary possibilities. The recipes in this chapter stand as delicious proof that you don't need artificial sweeteners, coloring agents, or ultra-processed ingredients to create meals that nourish both body and soul.

As I was recovering from my own heart surgery, these recipes became my culinary compass. They guided me toward healing while still providing the comfort and pleasure that food should bring. Whether I was building strength with protein-rich breakfasts, reducing inflammation with antioxidant-packed smoothies, or supporting my immune system with nutrient-dense dinners, these dishes made the healing process not just manageable, but enjoyable.

This collection represents a global tapestry of culinary wisdom, featuring contributions from talented chefs and nutrition experts from around the world who share a passion for clean, wholesome ingredients. From Mediterranean-inspired fish dishes to Asian-influenced salads, from Mexican-spiced bowls to European-style desserts, these recipes celebrate diverse culinary traditions while maintaining a steadfast commitment to whole food principles.

Every recipe has been carefully selected to support your healing journey. You'll find options rich in anti-inflammatory compounds, packed with essential vitamins and minerals, and designed to deliver the macronutrients your body needs for recovery. I have included icons to help you quickly identify the nutritional benefits of each dish, whether you're looking for high-protein meals, anti-inflammatory ingredients, or micronutrient-rich options.

Perhaps most importantly, these recipes are practical. They're designed for real life, with accessible ingredients and straightforward preparations. Healing doesn't mean spending hours in the kitchen or hunting down obscure ingredients. It means nourishing yourself with simple, wholesome foods that support your body's natural regenerative processes.

As you explore these recipes, I encourage you to approach them with a spirit of curiosity and flexibility. Feel free to adapt them to your preferences, dietary needs, and what's available seasonally. The true art of healthy cooking lies not in following recipes to the letter, but in understanding the principles of nourishing ingredients and making them work for your unique situation.

Let these recipes be your allies in healing, your guides to nourishment, and your invitation to discover that healthy eating can be one of life's great pleasures. From energizing breakfasts to comforting main dishes, from refreshing salads to satisfying sides, from guilt-free desserts to revitalizing tonics—each offering is a step on your path to wholeness.

Now, let's turn the page and begin a culinary journey that honors both the science of nutrition and the joy of eating well.

NOTE

If you have food sensitivities or allergies, we recommend consulting a healthcare professional or following an elimination program such as Whole30 before trying new recipes. Whenever possible, we encourage using organic ingredients—especially for items on the Environmental Working Group's "Dirty Dozen" list, which includes apples, blueberries, strawberries, spinach, kale, nectarines, peaches, cherries, pears, grapes, bell and hot peppers, and celery, as highlighted in Chapter 3. If organic options aren't available or affordable, focus on rinsing produce thoroughly and prioritizing fresh, seasonal ingredients when possible. We also recommend avoiding seed oils (such as canola, soybean, and sunflower oil) and ultra-processed ingredients to keep your meals as nourishing and clean as possible.

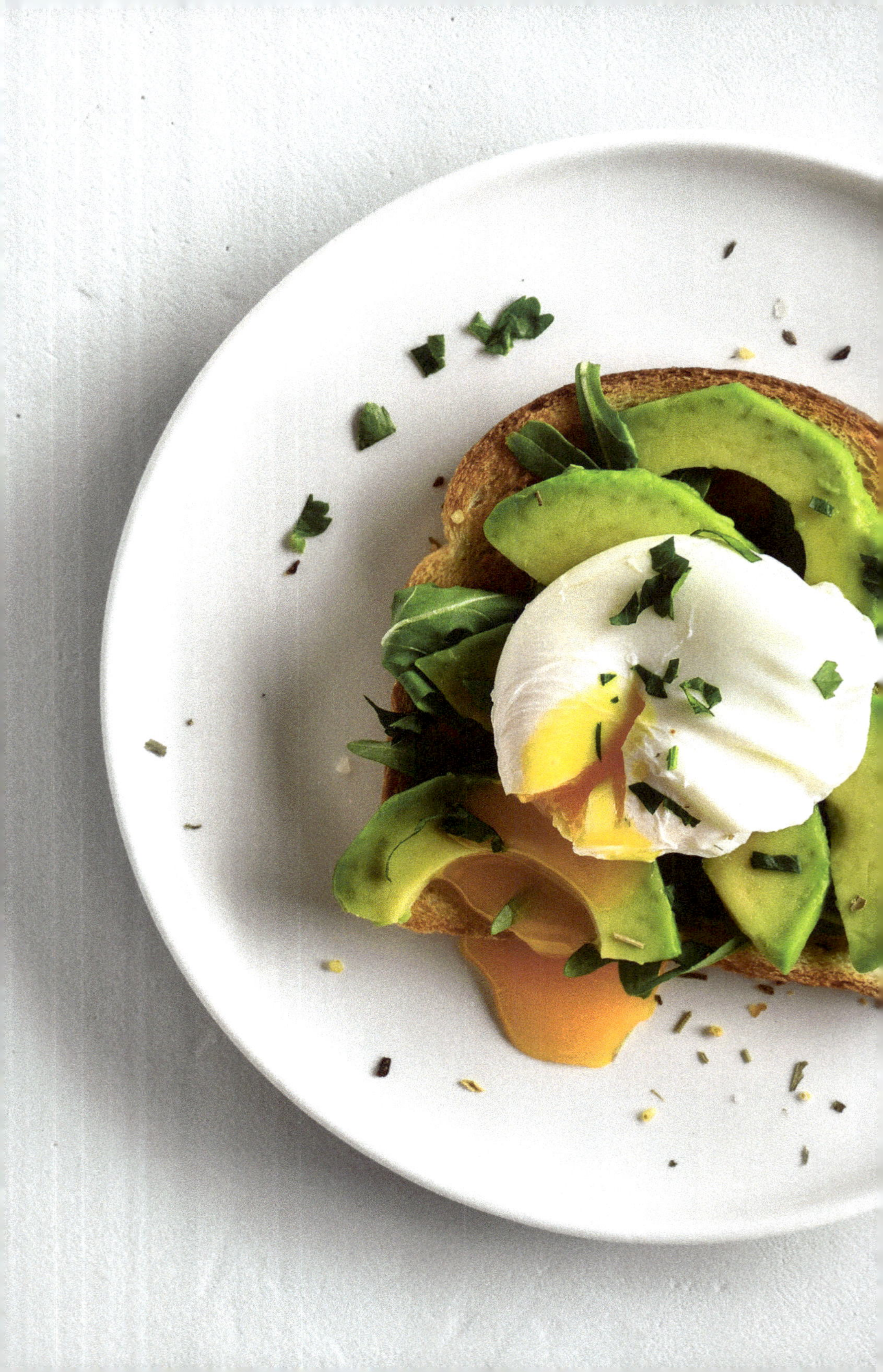

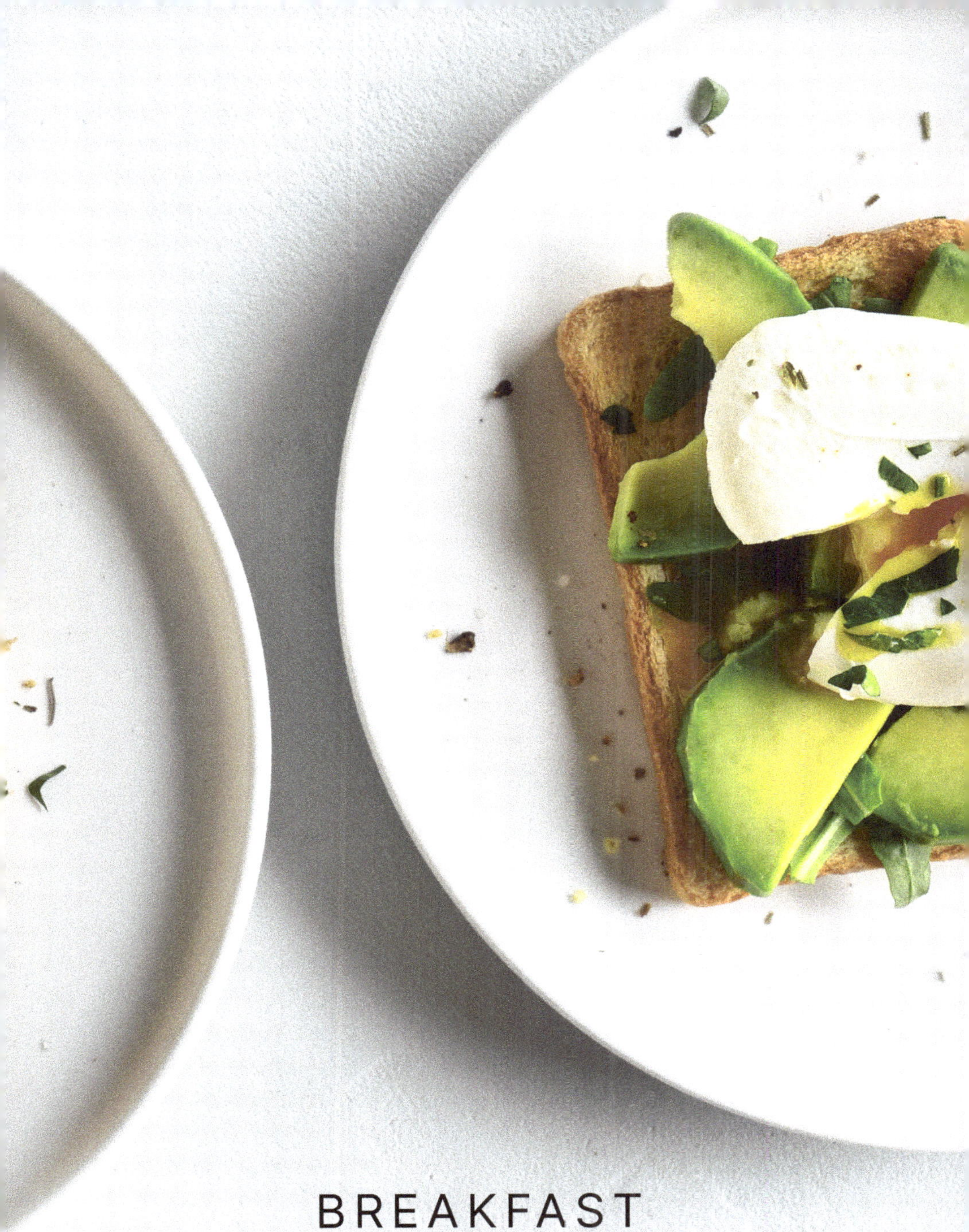

BREAKFAST

Blueberry Avocado Protein Bowl

Serves: 2 | *Prep Time: 10 minutes* | *Cook Time: 10 minutes*

This vibrant and nourishing bowl combines sweet and savory flavors with a punch of protein and healthy fats. While it might be counterintuitive to combine proteins like beef with something sweet, the clash in flavors actually makes this more interesting and unique. The flavors work together, in addition to the creamy feta, to offer a different twist on a protein bowl. Perfect for any time of day! This should be served immediately or stored in the refrigerator for up to two days.

INGREDIENTS

- ½ pound ground beef (grass-fed preferred)
- 1 Tbsp grass-fed butter
- 2 hard-boiled organic pasture-raised eggs, cut in half
- ½ cup organic blueberries
- ¼ cup organic feta cheese, crumbled
- 1 medium avocado, sliced
- 1 Tbsp raw honey (optional)
- ½ tsp ground cinnamon (optional)
- ¼ tsp flaky salt

INSTRUCTIONS

1. Heat a skillet over medium heat. Add the butter and ground beef and cook, breaking it apart with a spoon, until browned and cooked through (about 5–7 minutes).
2. Season with a pinch of flaky salt and divide the cooked ground beef evenly between two bowls.
3. Add the 2 hard-boiled eggs, ¼ cup blueberries, ½ avocado, and 2 Tbsp of crumbled feta to each bowl.
4. Drizzle each bowl with ½ a Tbsp of raw honey for a natural sweetness (optional) and sprinkle with a dash of ground cinnamon (optional).
5. Finish with a pinch of flaky salt to enhance the flavors.

Nutritional Facts (per serving):	
Disclaimer: *Nutritional values are estimates and may vary by ingredients and preparation.*	
Serves	2
Serving Size	1 bowl (approx. 400–450 g)
Calories	~620 kcal
Protein	35 g
Carbohydrates	17 g
Fiber	7 g
Sugars	8 g
Fats	44 g
Saturated Fat	15 g
Unsaturated Fat	27 g
Sodium	~480 mg
Vitamin A	~15% DV
Vitamin C	~20% DV
Calcium	~18% DV
Iron	~25% DV
Magnesium	~20% DV
Potassium	~700 mg

NOTES

Here are some optional additions to the bowl:

- A handful of leafy greens (spinach or arugula) for extra nutrients.
- Toasted nuts or seeds for added crunch.
- Swap ground beef with turkey or plant-based crumbles for variation.

Golden Oat Banana Muffins

Serves: 12 muffins | *Prep Time: 10 minutes* | *Cook Time: 20 minutes*

These muffins are the perfect breakfast or snack option. One thing I like to do when I am having a healthy treat is add a dollop of Greek yogurt or drizzle of nut butter on top. This adds a bit more protein and fat, making it slightly more filling. It is great on its own too, though. Bake these for the week and you have something to grab and snack on quickly. The potassium and slow carbs of the banana and oats, respectively, offer a sustaining fuel and nutrients. Most muffins are full of processed sugars and carbs from sugar, however, making them at home allows you to control what goes in, and these muffins are filled with nutritious goodness.

This recipe comes to us from Andrea Amatte, a viral recipe creator with millions of followers across the globe. She was kind enough to provide eight recipes for this book to give inspiration to those who want to make food that actually tastes great while still remaining healthy. You can find more of her work at @andrearecetas on Instagram.

INGREDIENTS

- 1 medium banana, mashed
- ¼ cup (60 ml) coconut oil, melted
- 1 tsp vanilla extract
- 3 large eggs
- 1 Tbsp plain yogurt
- 2½ cups (200 g) rolled oats
- 1 Tbsp baking powder
- 1 tsp ground cinnamon
- 1½ tsp monk fruit sweetener (or to taste)
- 1 pinch (about ⅛ tsp) ground ginger (optional)
- 1 tsp baking soda

DIRECTIONS

1. Preheat your oven to 350 degrees F (175 degrees C) and grease or line a muffin tin.
2. Mash the banana in a large bowl. Add the melted coconut oil and vanilla extract, then mix in the eggs. Beat everything together with a fork until smooth.
3. Stir in the yogurt until well combined.
4. In a separate bowl, combine the oats, baking powder, cinnamon, monk fruit sweetener, ginger (if using), and baking soda.

5. Fold the dry ingredients into the wet mixture using a spatula, mixing gently with circular motions until just combined.
6. Pour the batter evenly into the muffin tin.
7. Bake for 20 minutes or until a toothpick inserted in the center comes out clean.
8. Cool the muffins on a wire rack before serving.

Nutritional Facts (per serving):	
Disclaimer: *Nutritional values are estimates and may vary by ingredients and preparation.*	
Serves	**12**
Serving Size	**1 muffin**
Calories	**~140 kcal**
Protein	**4 g**
Carbohydrates	**13 g**
Fiber	**2 g**
Sugars	**2 g**
Fats	**8 g**
Saturated Fat	**5 g**
Unsaturated Fat	**3 g**
Sodium	**~120 mg**
Vitamin A	**~2% DV**
Vitamin C	**~3% DV**
Calcium	**~3% DV**
Iron	**~6% DV**
Magnesium	**~8% DV**
Potassium	**~150 mg**

Apple Pie Oats

Serves: 1 | Cook Time: 10 minutes

Oatmeal is a warm, comforting, and highly customizable dish that's perfect for your recovery journey. Packed with nutrients, oatmeal is an excellent source of fiber, protein, and essential vitamins that help keep you satisfied for hours, stabilize blood sugar levels, and support your overall health. It is ideal for those who may need softer foods during the initial days post-surgery, as oatmeal provides a gentle option that is easy on the stomach. Whether you prefer it warm in the morning or chilled and ready to grab from the fridge as overnight oats, this versatile meal can adapt to your lifestyle.

INGREDIENTS

- 1 Tbsp coconut oil
- 1 medium apple, diced
- Dash of cinnamon
- 1¼ cup water
- ½ cup oats
- 1 Tbsp nut butter of choice
- 1 Tbsp honey
- ⅓ cup granola (optional)

DIRECTIONS

1. On a flat pan, heat your coconut oil over medium-high heat.
2. Add your diced apples to the pan.
3. Sprinkle in some cinnamon to coat it and stir.
4. Cook until the apple is slightly browned and soft, about 5 minutes.
5. In a pot of water, heat your water until lightly boiling.
6. Stir in your oats; keep stirring continuously until it sets, about 5 minutes.
7. Plate your oats and add your honey, apple mixture, and optional toppings of granola and nut butter.

Nutritional Facts (per serving):	
Disclaimer: *Nutritional values are estimates and may vary by ingredients and preparation.*	
Serves	**1**
Serving Size	**1 bowl (approx. 300–350 g)**
Calories	**~390 kcal**
Protein	**7 g**
Carbohydrates	**45 g**
Fiber	**6 g**
Sugars	**16 g (from apple + honey)**
Fats	**19 g**
Saturated Fat	**7 g**
Unsaturated Fat	**12 g**
Sodium	**~20 mg**
Vitamin A	**~1% DV**
Vitamin C	**~8% DV**
Calcium	**~4% DV**
Iron	**~12% DV**
Magnesium	**~15% DV**
Potassium	**~350 mg**

NOTES

This recipe is for regular oats, but you can use any type you prefer (steel cut, regular, quick oats). Just make sure to adjust the cooking time to what is recommended on the package. Another tip add more water if you like oats with a more liquid-like texture.

Choco Chia Overnight Pudding

Serves: 1 | *Prep Time: 5 minutes* | *Cook Time: 3 hours or overnight*

Chia seeds are the underdog superfood. They don't get as much attention as they deserve, but are full of Omega-3s and fiber. Not to mention, two tablespoons has about five grams of protein. This pudding contains four tablespoons, so you will be getting a protein rich breakfast or snack that is relatively low in carbs. There is really no downside to chia seeds except patience as this pudding needs to be made overnight. However, you can also sprinkle them over oats, in smoothies, or on top of yogurt and eat them right away.

If you feel the need to switch up your regular morning oatmeal, this is a great alternative that you can customize any way you prefer. The trickiest part of the pudding is getting the liquid-to-chia seed balance just right. You want enough liquid for a pudding, but not so much that it turns into a soup. The below equation works out just right, but if you decide you want your pudding a bit more firm or liquidy, feel free to adjust to your liking.

INGREDIENTS

- 4 Tbsp chia seeds
- 1 cup coconut milk or almond milk
- 1 Tbsp cocoa powder
- 2 Tbsp honey or maple syrup, to taste
- ½ a banana
- 1 tsp cacao nibs, optional (they add a crunch)
- 1 scoop of protein powder

DIRECTIONS

1. In a bowl, mix chia seeds with coconut milk, cocoa powder, protein powder (optional), and maple syrup.
2. Stir well to prevent clumping. Refrigerate for at least 4 hours or overnight.
3. Serve with banana and cacao nibs on top.

Nutritional Facts (per serving):	
Disclaimer: *Nutritional values are estimates and may vary by ingredients and preparation.*	
Serves	1
Serving Size	1 bowl (approx. 250–300 g)
Calories	~410 kcal
Protein	20 g
Carbohydrates	32 g
Fiber	11 g
Sugars	13 g (from banana + honey/maple)
Fats	23 g
Saturated Fat	9 g
Unsaturated Fat	14 g
Sodium	~120 mg
Vitamin A	~2% DV
Vitamin C	~6% DV
Calcium	~25% DV
Iron	~15% DV
Magnesium	~30% DV
Potassium	~400 mg
Omega-3 (ALA)	~4,000 mg

Avocado Toast with a Twist

Servings: 1 | *Prep Time: 2 minutes* | *Cook Time: 10 minutes*

Once new and exotic, avocado toast has become a classic in the last few years. There are lots of interesting ways you can build your toast by customizing your toppings. You can make it spicy with sauces and pepper flakes, add crunchy toppings like toasted onion, or of course add eggs and other proteins on top. This recipe does the last opinion but offers a slightly different alternative than simple avocado with an egg on top. Instead, in this recipe you combine the ingredients into a spread. I really enjoy this version because the topping stays put, so you can eat the toast with your hands instead of a fork and knife, if that is something you prefer.

INGREDIENTS

- 2 boiled eggs, diced
- 1–2 slices of toast, toasted to your preference
- ½ small avocado, mashed
- 1 large scoop of cottage cheese
- Salt and pepper, to taste
- Sprinkle of paprika
- Fresh dill (optional but so good)

DIRECTIONS

1. Mix your eggs and avocado together with cottage cheese, salt and pepper, paprika and fresh dill.
2. Spread the mixture on your toast and enjoy.

Nutritional Facts (per serving):	
Disclaimer: *Nutritional values are estimates and may vary by ingredients and preparation.*	
Serves	1
Serving Size	1 toast with full topping (or split across 2 slices)
Calories	~360 kcal
Protein	20 g
Carbohydrates	22 g
Fiber	4 g
Sugars	2 g
Fats	21 g
Saturated Fat	6 g
Unsaturated Fat	15 g
Sodium	~390 mg
Vitamin A	~10% DV
Vitamin C	~6% DV
Calcium	~12% DV
Iron	~10% DV
Magnesium	~10% DV
Potassium	~450 mg
Omega-3 (ALA)	~4,000 mg

Gut Healthy Chia Oats

Servings: 1 | Prep Time: 5 minutes + overnight

Preparing meals in advance has great benefits for saving money, eating healthy, and saving time. It also helps you stick to a clean diet when the food is already prepared, removing one more task you have to do today, and one less decision to make. Overnight oats have become a sensation in recent years, and this recipe contains ingredients that can add additional benefits to an already healthy breakfast option. The fantastic aspect about this dish is that it is high in key nutrients like protein, complex carbs, fats, and vitamins and minerals.

INGREDIENTS

Base

- ½ cup oats
- ¼ cup chia seeds
- 2 scoops protein powder, such as Mendora (30g actual protein target)
- ½ cup milk, water or a mix
- 1 tsp flaxseed meal
- 2 Tbsp peanut butter

Toppings

- 2 Tbsp dark chocolate
- ½ tsp coconut oil
- Pumpkin seeds
- Coconut flakes
- Goji berries

DIRECTIONS

1. Mix oats, chia, protein, liquid of choice and stir well.
2. Add peanut butter and mix, it will harden in the fridge.
3. Add flaxseed meal and other toppings.
4. Microwave chocolate and coconut oil until runny together. Pour melted chocolate on top. Refrigerate overnight for best results.

Nutritional Facts (per serving):	
Disclaimer: *Nutritional values are estimates and may vary by ingredients and preparation.*	
Serves	1
Serving Size	1 bowl (approx. 350–400 g)
Calories	~540 kcal
Protein	32 g
Carbohydrates	34 g
Fiber	11 g
Sugars	7 g
Fats	31 g
Saturated Fat	7 g
Unsaturated Fat	24 g
Sodium	~180 mg
Vitamin A	~2% DV
Vitamin C	~2% DV
Calcium	~25% DV
Iron	~20% DV
Magnesium	~35% DV
Potassium	~500 mg
Omega-3 (ALA)	~4,500 mg

Protein Packed Low Carb Bagels

Servings: 4 bagels **|** *Prep Time: 10 minutes* **|** *Cook Time: 30 minutes*

Bagels are a classic breakfast and brunch option for a good reason. They are extremely versatile and filling. However, unless you are intentionally carb loading, the high amount of carbs can be slightly concerning for those who are interested in a leaner diet or a focus on higher protein intake. This option cuts the carbs down by substituting regular flour for the almond flour, which also makes it a safe choice for individuals avoiding gluten. Also, the secret ingredient of cottage cheese increases the protein significantly for a macro-friendly bagel option. As I indicated below, you can customize the seasonings sprinkled on top to suit your preference.

INGREDIENTS

- 2 cups of almond flour
- 1 cup cottage cheese
- 2 tsp baking powder
- 1 egg
- 1 tsp salt (optional)
- Sesame seeds or everything seasoning for topping (optional)

DIRECTIONS

1. Preheat your oven to 350 degrees F.
2. Mix almond flour, cottage cheese, baking powder, egg, and salt. If it's too dry, add a little warm water.
3. Add your preferred seasoning.
4. Knead the dough on a floured surface until smooth.
5. Form into a ball and divide into 4 pieces with a knife. Roll each into a ball, flatten slightly, and shape into bagels.
6. Brush with egg wash and sprinkle with seeds (optional).
7. Bake for 25–28 minutes until golden brown.

Nutritional Facts (per serving):	
Disclaimer: *Nutritional values are estimates and may vary by ingredients and preparation.*	
Serves	4
Serving Size	1 bagel
Calories	~280 kcal
Protein	16 g
Carbohydrates	7 g
Fiber	3 g
Sugars	1 g
Fats	22 g
Saturated Fat	4 g
Unsaturated Fat	18 g
Sodium	~320 mg
Vitamin A	~3% DV
Vitamin D	~4% DV
Calcium	~15% DV
Iron	~8% DV
Magnesium	~20% DV
Potassium	~200 mg

Sweet Potato Pancakes

Servings: 1–2 | *Prep Time: 5 minutes* | *Cook Time: 15 minutes*

People have been customizing pancakes for the last few years and it is so exciting to see how creative people are with each variation. This recipe uses the naturally sweet and delicious sweet potato, and you can add protein powder to give it more sweetness and protein content. Please note, the prep time above might take longer if you are baking or boiling your sweet potato. If you microwave it, about 5–8 minutes should be accurate. I recommend making a double batch to have something on hand for your next breakfast or sweet craving during the week.

INGREDIENTS

- 1 medium sweet potato
- 2 eggs
- 1 tsp cinnamon
- ½ Tbsp butter (optional)
- 1 tsp low-calorie sweetener (honey, Stevia, monk fruit extract)
- Drizzle with low-calorie syrup and/or nut butter (optional)

DIRECTIONS

1. Bake, boil, or microwave your sweet potato until the interior is soft. Once cool enough to handle, remove the skin.
2. Mash the interior of the sweet potato and mix with eggs, cinnamon, sweetener, and any optional ingredients.
3. Heat a nonstick pan or griddle over medium heat. Pour the batter and cook until bubbles form, then flip.
4. Stack, drizzle syrup, and enjoy your nutritious pancakes.

Nutritional Facts (per serving):	
Disclaimer: *Nutritional values are estimates and may vary by ingredients and preparation.*	
Serves	1
Serving Size	1 full stack (approx. 250–300 g)
Calories	~330 kcal
Protein	24 g
Carbohydrates	25 g
Fiber	4 g
Sugars	7 g (natural from sweet potato)
Fats	14 g
Saturated Fat	4 g
Unsaturated Fat	10 g
Sodium	~210 mg
Vitamin A	~300% DV
Vitamin C	~10% DV
Calcium	~10% DV
Iron	~12% DV
Magnesium	~15% DV
Potassium	~500 mg

Nut and Seed Granola Bars

Servings: about 12 bars | *Prep Time: 10 minutes* | *Cook Time: 20–30 minutes*

Granola bars are the ultimate grab and go food, but most store-purchased options come with preservatives, sweeteners, or fillers. This recipe allows you to take control of what you put in your bars. That way, if you feel the call of hunger you have something quick and healthy on hand to tide you over until your next meal. With a variety of nuts and seeds, you have a fantastic micronutrient rich snack here. It is perfect for meal prepping before the week starts. You can even save half the batch for the week ahead, and freeze the other half if you prefer. To thaw, you can leave them at room temperature for at least an hour, or gently defrost them in the microwave for a few minutes.

INGREDIENTS

- 1 cup almonds
- 2 cups cashews
- 1 cup pumpkin seeds
- 1 cup sunflower seeds
- ½ cup chia seeds
- ½ cup maple syrup
- 1 cup dark chocolate (optional)
- 1–2 tsp coconut oil (optional)

DIRECTIONS

1. Prepare a parchment-lined baking sheet and preheat your oven to 350 degrees F.
2. Mix all ingredients together in a bowl, making sure the syrup is coated evenly around.
3. Spread your mixture on the parchment-lined sheet and bake for 25–30 minutes.
4. Let cool completely before cutting into 12 or more (depending how big or small you want them).
5. Put your dark chocolate in a microwave-safe bowl with some coconut oil. Make sure the microwave is set to medium heat and stir it every 15–20 seconds to make sure it does not burn.
6. Using two forks or tongs, coat one side of your bars with the chocolate and place on a parchment lined sheet to cool and harden. Drizzle the other sides afterwards as well.

Nutritional Facts (per serving):	
Disclaimer: *Nutritional values are estimates and may vary by ingredients and preparation.*	
Serves	12
Serving Size	1 bar (approx. 60–70 g)
Calories	~330 kcal
Protein	8 g
Carbohydrates	20 g
Fiber	5 g
Sugars	9 g (from maple syrup and chocolate)
Fats	24 g
Saturated Fat	6 g
Unsaturated Fat	18 g
Sodium	~5 mg
Vitamin E	~25% DV
Magnesium	~30% DV
Iron	~15% DV
Zinc	~20% DV
Potassium	~250 mg
Omega-3 (ALA)	~2,500 mg

Tiramisu Chia Pudding

Servings: 1 **|** *Prep Time: 5 minutes active, 4 hours/overnight to soak*

Tiramisu is a classic Italian dessert and one of my favorites, but the original recipe uses a lot of mascarpone cheese and sugar. This recipe offers a healthier and lower-fat, higher-protein option that you can have for breakfast or dessert, as often as you desire. Isabella is not only a nutritionist but a content creator who helps people create a lifestyle focused fitness program. If you have not tried chia seeds before, just note that they take a bit of time to soak and form into a pudding texture, but are well worth it as long as you prepare in advance. Like many of the recipes in this book, this once can easily be doubled or tripled in different containers, ready to consume. Also to note, since it is a pudding, the texture is of course soft enough for the earlier stages of your recovery. The protein, healthy fat, and fiber in chia seeds makes this a health staple.

INGREDIENTS

- 3 Tbsp chia seeds
- 1 cup high protein yogurt
- ¼ cup (1 shot) of coffee
- 2 tsp of maple syrup
- 1 Tbsp cacao powder

DIRECTIONS

1. Mix the chia seeds, yogurt, coffee and sweetener together in a Tupperware. Stir thoroughly to ensure the chia seeds are evenly distributed.
2. Cover the Tupperware and place it in the fridge for at least 4 hours or overnight. This allows the chia seeds to absorb the liquid and thicken into a pudding-like consistency.
3. Before serving, sprinkle with a generous amount of cacao powder and enjoy.

Nutritional Facts (per serving):	
Disclaimer: *Nutritional values are estimates and may vary by ingredients and preparation.*	
Serves	1
Serving Size	1 jar/bowl (approx. 250–300 g)
Calories	~290 kcal
Protein	22 g
Carbohydrates	16 g
Fiber	10 g
Sugars	6 g
Fats	13 g
Saturated Fat	4 g
Unsaturated Fat	9 g
Sodium	~90 mg
Calcium	~25% DV
Iron	~10% DV
Magnesium	~20% DV
Potassium	~300 mg
Omega-3 (ALA)	~3,000 mg

NOTE

The coffee in the ingredients means a shot of espresso or shot of coffee made in the Cuban and Italian style coffee maker, not American drip coffee which is too diluted for this recipe.

Homemade Pumpkin Granola

Servings: 10 | *Prep Time: 10 minutes* | *Cook Time: 25 minutes*

If you go crazy for pumpkin-spiced foods and drinks in the fall, you have found an easy recipe here that you can make year round. Since the recipes only used pumpkin seeds and pumpkin spice, you don't need to worry about purchasing seasonal pumpkin produce. However, it hits the spot when you are in the mood for something that tastes like fall. If you like to eat granola by itself, go crazy. But the way I recommend eating it is by adding it to some milk and eating it like cereal, or sprinkling it on top of yogurt to make a parfait.

This granola recipe is provided for this book by holistic chef Elizabeth Leigh Mandelbaum. Her focus on clean and simple ingredients is excellent for a whole-food focused diet like we have been talking about throughout the book. I highly recommend you try her recipes in this book, the ones posted on social media, and in her cookbook *Plated.*

INGREDIENTS

- 3 cups organic oats
- 3 Tbsp chia seeds
- ⅓ cup pumpkin seeds
- ½ cup maple syrup
- ¾ cup coconut oil
- ½ tsp cinnamon
- ½ tsp pumpkin spice

DIRECTIONS

1. Preheat the oven to 350 degrees F.
2. In a mixing bowl, mix together all of the ingredients above and stir until fully combined. Then spread the mixture onto a lined baking sheet.
3. Bake for 20–25 minutes. Let it cool, store in a glass jar sealed tightly.
4. Place ½ cup of your favorite yogurt in a bowl then top with the most delicious granola. Enjoy!

Nutritional Facts (per serving):	
Disclaimer: *Nutritional values are estimates and may vary by ingredients and preparation.*	
Serves	10
Serving Size	~½ cup (approx. 45–50 g)
Calories	~240 kcal
Protein	4 g
Carbohydrates	23 g
Fiber	3 g
Sugars	7 g (from maple syrup)
Fats	15 g
Saturated Fat	10 g
Unsaturated Fat	5 g
Sodium	~5 mg
Iron	~10% DV
Magnesium	~20% DV
Zinc	~12% DV
Potassium	~150 mg

Crescent Egg Tortilla

Serves: 1 | *Cook time: 10 minutes*

There is nothing more satisfying than eggs for breakfast. They are one of the most versatile foods; chefs have found hundreds of creative ways to cook them. While I would never turn down a traditional egg scramble, sometimes it's nice to do something a little different. This dish is simple yet offers a little more variety for breakfast. You can cook and assemble it in just one pan, and it includes protein, carbs, and some veggies to boot.

INGREDIENTS

- 1 Tbsp olive oil
- 1 tortilla of choice
- 2 eggs
- Salad greens
- ½ Roma tomato
- ¼ cup shredded cheese of choice

DIRECTIONS

1. Heat a medium-sized pan over medium heat. Coat with olive oil.
2. Whisk your eggs in a bowl with some salt and pepper and pour it in the pan in an even layer. Allow to cook for a minute.
3. Place your tortilla in the pan right on top of your eggs while they are still mostly liquid.
4. Let your eggs cook until firm and flip over the tortilla on its uncooked side.
5. While that side toasts, add your tomato, greens, and shredded cheese on top of the egg. Fold in half and allow the cheese to melt it together.
6. Serve and enjoy.

Nutritional Facts (per serving):	
Disclaimer: *Nutritional values are estimates and may vary by ingredients and preparation.*	
Serves	1
Serving Size	1 full wrap (~250–275 g)
Calories	~370 kcal
Protein	22 g
Carbohydrates	20 g
Fiber	3 g
Sugars	2 g (from tomato and greens)
Fats	24 g
Saturated Fat	10 g
Unsaturated Fat	14 g
Sodium	~480 mg
Vitamin A	~35% DV
Vitamin C	~20% DV
Calcium	~25% DV
Iron	~15% DV
Magnesium	~10% DV
Potassium	~350 mg
Antioxidants	Moderate to high (from tomato, greens, and eggs)

Super Simple High-Protein Quiche

Serves: 2–4 **|** *Cook time: 10 minutes*

I have fond memories of eating quiches during special occasions, however, given the effort they usually take to cook—in addition to the high fat content—they are not practical to eat on a regular basis. This quiche is luckily not your everyday quiche. Starting off, we swap the butter-heavy crust for a light and low-fat tortilla wrap. They even have wrap options that are made with almond flour, bean flour, rice flour, the list goes on. You can choose, so long as it is a large size. Next, we swap the heavy cream for some cottage cheese which typically has lower fat and higher protein content. By adding some veggies as well, we add in some micronutrients to make a balanced dish. Another selling point of this quiche is you can make and assemble it in just one pan for very little kitchen clean up.

INGREDIENTS

- 3 eggs
- ⅓ cup cottage cheese
- ⅕ cup diced red peppers
- 1–1½ cups spinach
- ½ cup low-fat shredded mozzarella cheese
- Salt and pepper to taste
- Low-fat tortilla wrap

DIRECTIONS

1. Preheat your oven to 350 degrees F and place the wrap in a round 8-inch diameter oven-safe pan.
2. Use your hands to settle it to the bottom part of the pan—the sides will get naturally wavy.
3. Once the shape holds, in a separate bowl, add your eggs, cottage cheese, veggies, and seasonings. Mix together and pour into the pan.
4. Cook for 20 to 25 minutes.

Nutritional Facts (per serving):	
Disclaimer: *Nutritional values are estimates and may vary by ingredients and preparation.*	
Serves	2
Serving Size	~1 portion (~200–225 g)
Calories	~210 kcal
Protein	22 g
Carbohydrates	4 g
Fiber	1 g
Sugars	2 g (naturally from peppers and dairy)
Fats	11 g
Saturated Fat	4.5 g
Unsaturated Fat	6.5 g
Sodium	~360 mg (varies by cheese and added salt)
Vitamin A	~60% DV
Vitamin C	~45% DV
Calcium	~25% DV
Iron	~12% DV
Magnesium	~10% DV
Potassium	~450 mg
Antioxidants	High (from spinach, red peppers, and eggs)

Pesto Feta Omelette

Serves: 1 | *Cook time: 10 minutes*

Start your morning with a delicious and protein-packed twist on a classic breakfast—an egg omelette infused with rich, flavorful pesto sauce. This unique recipe takes the traditional basil pesto, typically used in pasta and sandwiches, and blends it seamlessly into a fluffy, golden omelette. Not only does it provide a boost of protein to keep you energized throughout the day, but it also delivers a burst of fresh, herby goodness in every bite. The creamy texture of the eggs pairs perfectly with the nutty, garlicky essence of the pesto, making it a gourmet yet simple dish to prepare. Whether you're looking for a quick weekday breakfast or a special weekend treat, this pesto omelette is a must-try for any food lover!

INGREDIENTS

- ⅓ cup of shredded cheese
- 2 medium eggs
- 1 oz pesto sauce (store bought or homemade)
- 1 oz feta cheese
- 1 Roma tomato
- Olive oil to cook
- Salt and pepper to taste

DIRECTIONS

1. Drizzle some olive oil on a small pan over medium heat.
2. Sprinkle in your shredded cheese to coat the bottom of the pan.
3. Whisk and season your eggs. Add them in the pan.
4. Once the eggs are slightly firm, add in your pesto sauce in a line down the middle. Then, put your feta and sliced tomato directly on top.
5. Allow to cook until the bottom of the egg mixture is solid. Then, fold both sides in together to cover the toppings like a blanket. Allow to cook fully and serve.

Nutritional Facts (per serving):	
Disclaimer: *Nutritional values are estimates and may vary by ingredients and preparation.*	
Serves	1
Serving Size	1 plate (~250 g)
Calories	~390 kcal
Protein	23 g
Carbohydrates	6 g
Fiber	1.5 g
Sugars	3 g (from tomato)
Fats	31 g
Saturated Fat	10 g
Unsaturated Fat	21 g
Sodium	~500 mg (depends on feta, pesto, and added salt)
Vitamin A	~30% DV
Vitamin C	~20% DV
Calcium	~25% DV
Iron	~10% DV
Magnesium	~8% DV
Potassium	~400 mg
Antioxidants	Moderate to high (from tomato, olive oil, pesto herbs, and eggs)

Smoked Salmon Over Crispy Potatoes

Serves: 1 pie, 8 slices | *Cook time: 10 minutes*

Elevate your breakfast with a delicious and nutrient-rich combination of smoked salmon served over a bed of crispy baked potatoes. This high-protein dish is packed with essential omega-3 fatty acids, which support heart and brain health, while the potatoes provide a satisfying source of fiber and complex carbohydrates for lasting energy. The smoky, savory flavor of the salmon pairs beautifully with the golden, crunchy potatoes, creating a balanced and flavorful meal. Rich in vitamins B12 and D, this breakfast option helps support metabolism and immune function, making it as nutritious as it is delicious. Whether you're fueling up for a busy day or indulging in a weekend brunch, this dish is a perfect blend of taste and health benefits.

INGREDIENTS

- 8 small potatoes (about 200 grams), boiled
- 1 cup Greek yogurt
- ½ a lemon (juice and zest to garnish)
- 1 bulb of garlic, minced
- 4–6 oz smoked salmon
- Handful of arugula for topping
- Drizzle of olive oil for topping
- Salt and pepper for topping

DIRECTIONS

1. Preheat your oven to 350 degrees F and prepare a parchment-lined baking sheet.
2. Boil your potatoes (about 20 minutes) and smash them over the baking sheet and form them into a sort of round base.
3. Add desired seasonings and bake for about 30 minutes until the top is crispy brown.
4. While waiting, mix your yogurt, lemon juice, and garlic together.
5. Remove potato base from oven, allow to cool, and smooth the yogurt on top. Then add your salmon.
6. Garnish with arugula, lemon zest, salt and pepper, and olive oil. Enjoy!

Nutritional Facts (per serving):	
Disclaimer: *Nutritional values are estimates and may vary by ingredients and preparation.*	
Serves	**8**
Serving Size	**1 slice (~130–150 g)**
Calories	**~160 kcal**
Protein	**10 g**
Carbohydrates	**10 g**
Fiber	**1.5 g**
Sugars	**1 g (naturally from yogurt and potato)**
Fats	**9 g**
Saturated Fat	**2 g**
Unsaturated Fat	**7 g**
Sodium	**~280 mg (mainly from smoked salmon and added salt)**
Vitamin A	**~6% DV**
Vitamin C	**~15% DV**
Calcium	**~8% DV**
Iron	**~6% DV**
Magnesium	**~6% DV**
Potassium	**~400 mg**
Antioxidants	**Moderate to high (from arugula, lemon, garlic, and**

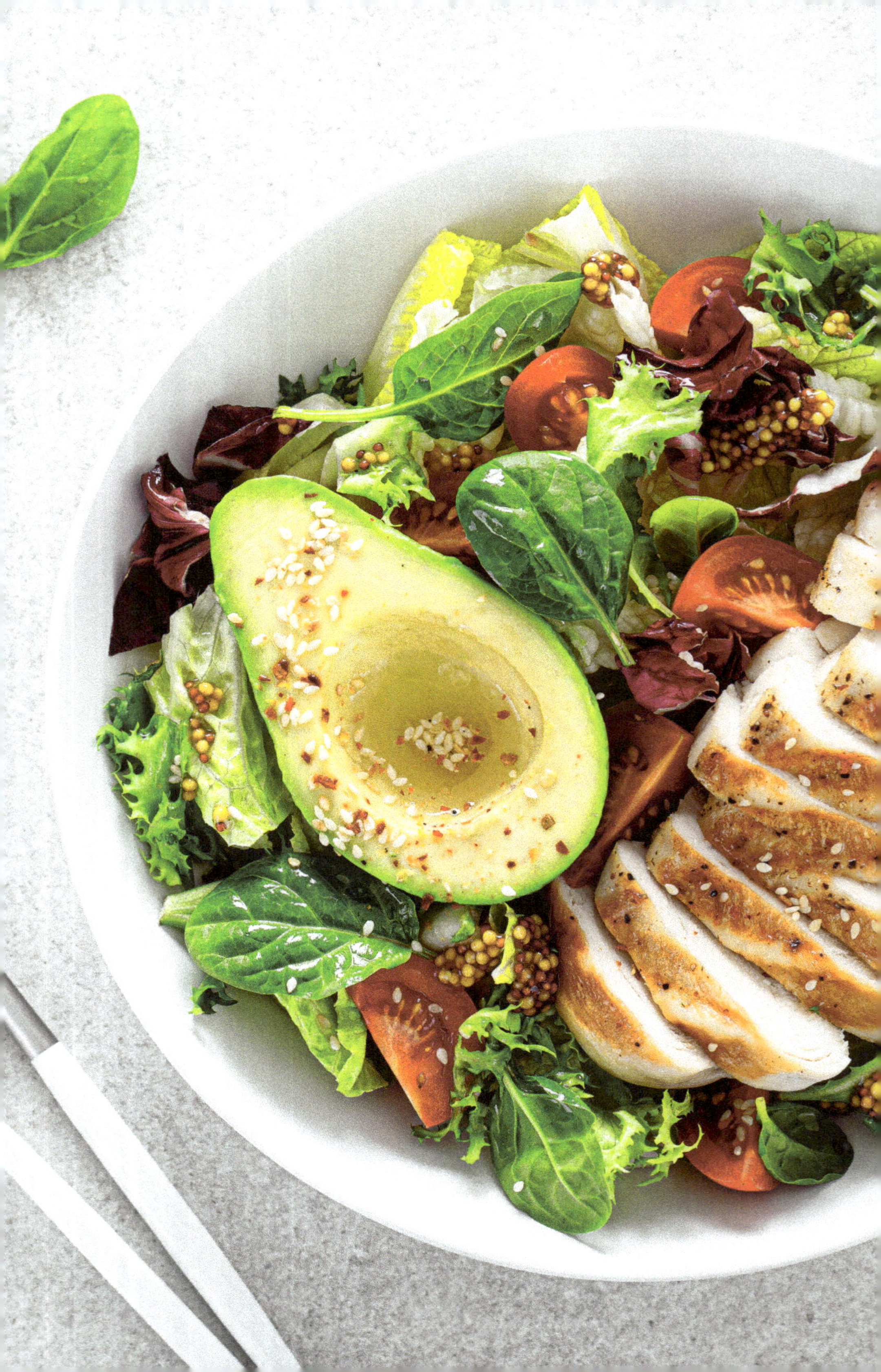

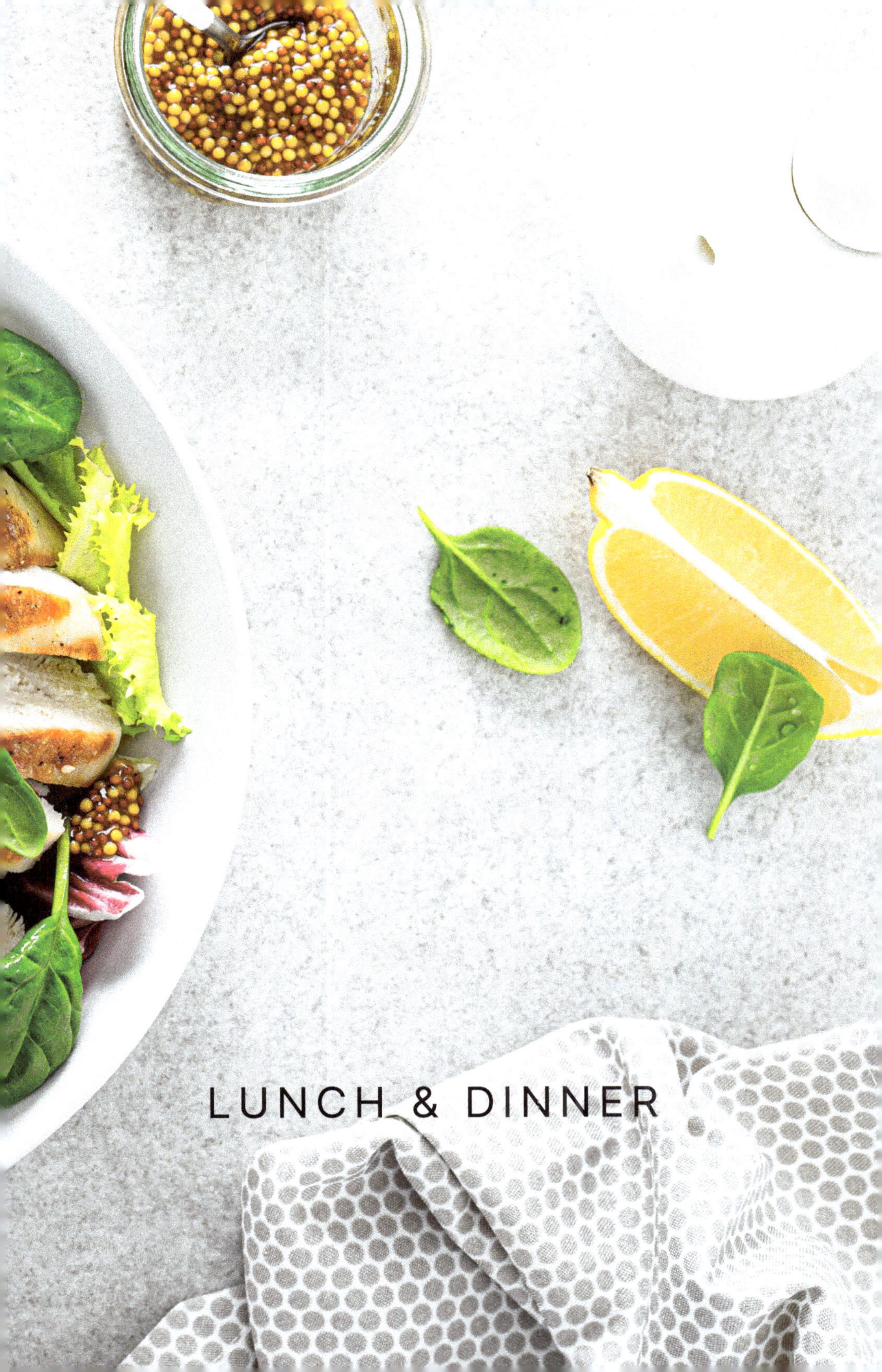

LUNCH & DINNER

Nourishing Chicken and Kale Soup

Serves: 2 | *Prep Time: 10 minutes* | *Cook Time: 40 minutes*

This wholesome soup is not only filled with tender, succulent chunks of chicken that practically melt in your mouth, but it also boasts a variety of vibrant vegetables that can be tailored to suit your preferences or whatever you have on hand. The addition of kale packs a nutrient dense punch. Ideal for those needing softer foods during the initial days post-surgery, this chicken and vegetable soup provides a hearty yet gentle option for your stomach.

INGREDIENTS

- 3 large carrots
- 2 stalks of celery
- 2 large potatoes
- 1 small white onion, diced
- 2 Tbsp olive oil
- 7 oz / 200 grams of chicken or beef
- Spices: 1 tsp garlic powder, 1 tsp salt, 2 bay leaves, 1 bouillon cube
- 4–6 cups bone broth
- 1 cup kale, thinly sliced

DIRECTIONS

1. Chop all your veggies, potatoes; slice chicken thinly and set all aside.
2. Pour your olive oil in a pot over medium heat. Add your onion and sauté until fragrant.
3. Place chicken slices in; add spices and some salt.
4. Add your potatoes and veggies, except the kale.
5. Add bone broth and top it off with about 3–4 more cups of regular water, so that it is entirely covered. Cover the saucepan so that it is closed airtight.
6. Simmer on low heat for 30 minutes. Taste it, adjust spices if needed.
7. Add your kale, then simmer for 5 minutes.
8. Serve and top it off with some cracked pepper.

Nutritional Facts (per serving):	
Disclaimer: *Nutritional values are estimates and may vary by ingredients and preparation.*	
Serves	2
Serving Size	~1 large bowl (~500–600 g)
Calories	~490 kcal
Protein	28 g
Carbohydrates	35 g
Fiber	6 g
Sugars	7 g (from carrots, onion, and potato)
Fats	26 g
Saturated Fat	6 g
Unsaturated Fat	20 g
Sodium	~850 mg (from broth, bouillon, and added salt)
Vitamin A	~220% DV
Vitamin C	~45% DV
Calcium	~12% DV
Iron	~20% DV
Magnesium	~18% DV
Potassium	~1,200 mg
Antioxidants	High (from kale, olive oil, carrots, onion, and spices)

NOTES

Feel free to modify the recipe by incorporating your favorite vegetables. This flexibility not only allows you to create a personalized meal that suits your taste but also ensures that you're getting a healthy variety of nutrients as you heal.

Immunity Carrot Ginger Soup

Servings: 2–4 | *Prep Time: 10 minutes* | *Cook Time: 45 minutes*

Soups are a fantastic way to get a variety of nutrients while being gentle on the stomach. This soup also has the superpower of being good for your immune system and easy to make. With only five ingredients (salt and pepper optional), it is one of the quickest soups you'll probably ever make.

INGREDIENTS

- 2 cups / 500g carrots, roughly chopped
- 2 red onions roughly chopped
- 1 thumb-sized piece of ginger, peeled
- 1 Tbsp turmeric
- 1 vegetable stock cube

DIRECTIONS

1. Turn the oven to 400 degrees F. Prepare a parchment-lined baking sheet.
2. Add your carrots, onions, and ginger to the baking sheet.
3. Drizzle a little oil over the top and then add the turmeric, give everything a good tumble together, season if you wish, and cover with foil.
4. Place the tray in the oven for 35–45 minutes then remove and add the vegetables to a food processor along with the cube and a little water to loosen then blitz until smooth.
5. Pour the mixture into a saucepan with 500ml of water and bring to a gentle simmer. Check for seasoning and you're done!

Nutritional Facts (per serving):	
Disclaimer: *Nutritional values are estimates and may vary by ingredients and preparation.*	
Serves	4
Serving Size	1 bowl (~300–350 ml)
Calories	~100 kcal
Protein	2 g
Carbohydrates	18 g
Fiber	5 g
Sugars	8 g (natural from carrots and onions)
Fats	3 g
Saturated Fat	0.4 g
Unsaturated Fat	2.6 g
Sodium	~400 mg (from stock cube)
Vitamin A	~280% DV
Vitamin C	~12% DV
Calcium	~5% DV
Iron	~6% DV
Magnesium	~8% DV
Potassium	~600 mg

Lentil Veggie Stew

Serves: 4–6 | *Prep Time: 10 minutes* | *Cook time: 2 hours simmering*

This stew is a weekly standard in my home. It is hearty, nourishing, and made with wholesome ingredients like lentils, carrots, and celery. Packed with plant-based protein, fiber, and essential vitamins, it supports immune health and promotes steady energy—perfect for healing. The lentils offer iron and protein to aid tissue repair, while the veggies provide antioxidants and anti-inflammatory nutrients. This comforting stew is ideal for recovery after surgery, giving your body the fuel it needs to rebuild and restore.

INGREDIENTS

- 2 cups lentils
- 4 carrots
- 1 medium onion
- 4 qts. water
- 2 bouillon cubes
- 4 sticks celery
- 2 tsp mixed herb powder
- ½ tsp salt, more to taste
- 1 tsp thyme
- 1 Tablespoon lemon juice
- 1 Tablespoon olive oil

DIRECTIONS

1. Soak lentils overnight in room temperature water.
2. When ready to cook, strain the lentils, disposing of the water used to soak them.
3. Pour 4 quarts of fresh water in a pot. Add salt and stew the lentils very gently for 1 hour, taking off any scum that rises to the surface.
4. Wash the vegetables well, slice them, and add to the soup.
5. Stew for 1 hour more. Then rub through a sieve, or not, as preferred.
6. Add the lemon juice, herb powder, and olive oil, and serve.

Nutritional Facts (per serving):	
Disclaimer: *Nutritional values are estimates and may vary by ingredients and preparation.*	
Serves	6
Serving Size	1 large bowl (~400–450 ml)
Calories	~280 kcal
Protein	17 g
Carbohydrates	34 g
Fiber	14 g
Sugars	4 g
Fats	5 g
Saturated Fat	0.7 g
Unsaturated Fat	4.3 g
Sodium	~420 mg
Vitamin A	~110% DV
Vitamin C	~15% DV
Calcium	~6% DV
Iron	~25% DV
Magnesium	~20% DV
Potassium	~600 mg

Perla's Perfect Salmon

Servings: 3–4 | Prep Time: 5 minutes | Cook Time: 10–20 minutes

Salmon is a holy grail food for many health reasons. It has healthy omega-3 fats that could reduce inflammation, lower blood pressure, and improve your heart health. If you factor in the wonderful protein content and the numerous vitamins and antioxidants, you have tons of nourishment in just one fish. Also, it is versatile. There are many ways you can have salmon: smoked, oven or pan roasted, steamed, made into salmon patties, sushi, the list goes on.

This and the next three delicious recipes are provided courtesy of Ilana Muhlstein, author of *Love the Food That Loves You Back* (Mango Publishing), which is a fantastic clean eating cookbook you should check out next. Ilana is a Registered Dietitian Nutritionist and offers amazing meal inspiration and nutrition guidance. You can find out more about her work by booking a private session with her, purchasing her cookbook, and following her on social media at @ilanamuhlsteinrd.

INGREDIENTS

- 1 lb salmon
- 1½ tsp olive oil
- ½ tsp garlic powder
- ½ tsp salt
- 1 tsp dry dill
- Lemon slices for serving

DIRECTIONS

1. Preheat the oven to 400 degrees F.
2. Line a baking sheet with parchment paper.
3. Place salmon on the baking sheet skin side down.
4. Rub the flesh of the salmon with the olive oil.
5. Sprinkle an even layer of garlic powder, salt, and dill over the salmon.
6. Bake for 17 to 19 minutes. If using an air fryer, cook at 400 degrees F for 7 to 10 minutes.
7. It is great served warm, cold, or at room temperature.

Nutritional Facts (per serving):	
Disclaimer: *Nutritional values are estimates and may vary by ingredients and preparation.*	
Serves	4
Serving Size	~4 oz salmon (~113 g cooked)
Calories	~185 kcal
Protein	20 g
Carbohydrates	0 g
Fiber	0 g
Sugars	0 g
Fats	11 g
Saturated Fat	2 g
Unsaturated Fat	9 g
Sodium	~215 mg
Vitamin A	~3% DV
Vitamin C	~2% DV (from lemon slices if used)
Calcium	~1% DV
Iron	~3% DV
Magnesium	~6% DV
Potassium	~425 mg
Antioxidants	Moderate (from garlic, dill, and olive oil)

Spaghetti Squash Cacio E Pepe

Servings: 2–4 | *Cook Time: 10 minutes*

Italian cuisine is a favorite of mine and life wouldn't be complete without some of it in my diet. This is another delicious creation from nutritionist Ilana Muhlstein that offers a healthier low-carb twist to Cacio e Pepe (Cheese and Pepper), a classic Italian recipe. By using squash instead of pasta, we add more nutrients and fiber to our plate. If you're not sure how to make the spaghetti part of this, look over to my note below.

This recipe is also provided for this book courtesy of Registered Dietitian Nutritionist Ilana Muhlstein, author of *Love the Food That Loves You Back*. You can find out more about her work by booking a private session with her, purchasing her cookbook, and following her on social media at @ilanamuhlsteinrd.

INGREDIENTS

- 6 cups cooked spaghetti squash
- ¼–½ cup aquafaba, the reserved liquid from a can of chickpeas (a.k.a. garbanzo beans) or a cornstarch slurry made by mixing 4 Tbsp cold water with 2 Tbsp cornstarch
- ½ cup Parmesan cheese, grated
- ½ tsp black pepper

DIRECTIONS

1. Toast black pepper in a large saucepan over low to medium heat for 1 to 2 minutes, or until fragrant.
2. Add Parmesan cheese and aquafaba or cornstarch slurry to the large saucepan and stir vigorously until well combined.
3. Once evenly mixed into a thick sauce, add in your spaghetti squash.
4. Stir continuously until it's evenly mixed.
5. Garnish with fresh basil (optional).

Nutritional Facts (per serving):	
Disclaimer: *Nutritional values are estimates and may vary by ingredients and preparation.*	
Serves	4
Serving Size	~1½ cups (~220–250 g)
Calories	~115 kcal
Protein	6 g
Carbohydrates	15 g
Fiber	3 g
Sugars	5 g (naturally from squash)
Fats	4.5 g
Saturated Fat	2.5 g
Unsaturated Fat	2 g
Sodium	~270 mg
Vitamin A	~6% DV
Vitamin C	~10% DV
Calcium	~15% DV
Iron	~4% DV
Magnesium	~10% DV
Potassium	~400 mg
Antioxidants	Moderate (especially if garnished with basil)

NOTE

To get the "spaghetti" part, cut a squash in half and scoop out the seeds. Season with salt and pepper and roast it facedown in the oven for about 30–40 minutes. Using a fork, shred the soft inner part into spaghetti.

Mushroom Cap Pizzas

Servings: 1–2 | *Cook Time: 20 minutes*

What is life without a little fun? Pizza is the ultimate fun food, but with the heavy fat and simple carbs typically in pizzas, it is not the ideal dish for a healing, anti-inflammatory diet. Luckily, there are many fun comfort foods we can make into healthy versions. As the title suggests, this pizza recipe is made on top of the caps of large mushrooms. This makes them a great solo meal or shared snack with an excellent source of vitamins, minerals, and antioxidants.

This recipe is also provided for this book courtesy of Registered Dietitian Nutritionist Ilana Muhlstein, author of *Love the Food That Loves You Back*. You can find out more about her work by booking a private session with her, purchasing her cookbook, and following her on social media at @ilanamuhlsteinrd.

INGREDIENTS

- 2 large mushroom caps, cleaned
- ¼ cup pizza or marinara sauce
- ⅓ cup part skim mozzarella cheese, grated
- Garlic powder and red chili flakes to taste
- Additional toppings of your choice (optional)

DIRECTIONS

1. Line a baking sheet with parchment paper and spray with oil.
2. Preheat the oven to 400 degrees F.
3. Bake 2 mushroom caps, gills side up, for 5 minutes.
4. Carefully remove the pan from the oven and blot away the excess liquid.
5. Top the mushroom caps evenly with sauce and cheese, then bake for another 10 minutes or until the cheese is bubbly.

Nutritional Facts (per serving):	
Disclaimer: *Nutritional values are estimates and may vary by ingredients and preparation.*	
Serves	2
Serving Size	1 stuffed mushroom cap (~150–170 g)
Calories	~110 kcal
Protein	8 g
Carbohydrates	8 g
Fiber	2 g
Sugars	4 g (from marinara sauce and mushrooms)
Fats	6 g
Saturated Fat	3.5 g
Unsaturated Fat	2.5 g
Sodium	~300 mg
Vitamin A	~6% DV
Vitamin C	~4% DV
Calcium	~12% DV
Iron	~4% DV
Magnesium	~5% DV
Potassium	~400 mg
Antioxidants	Moderate to high (especially from mushrooms, marinara, and chili flakes)

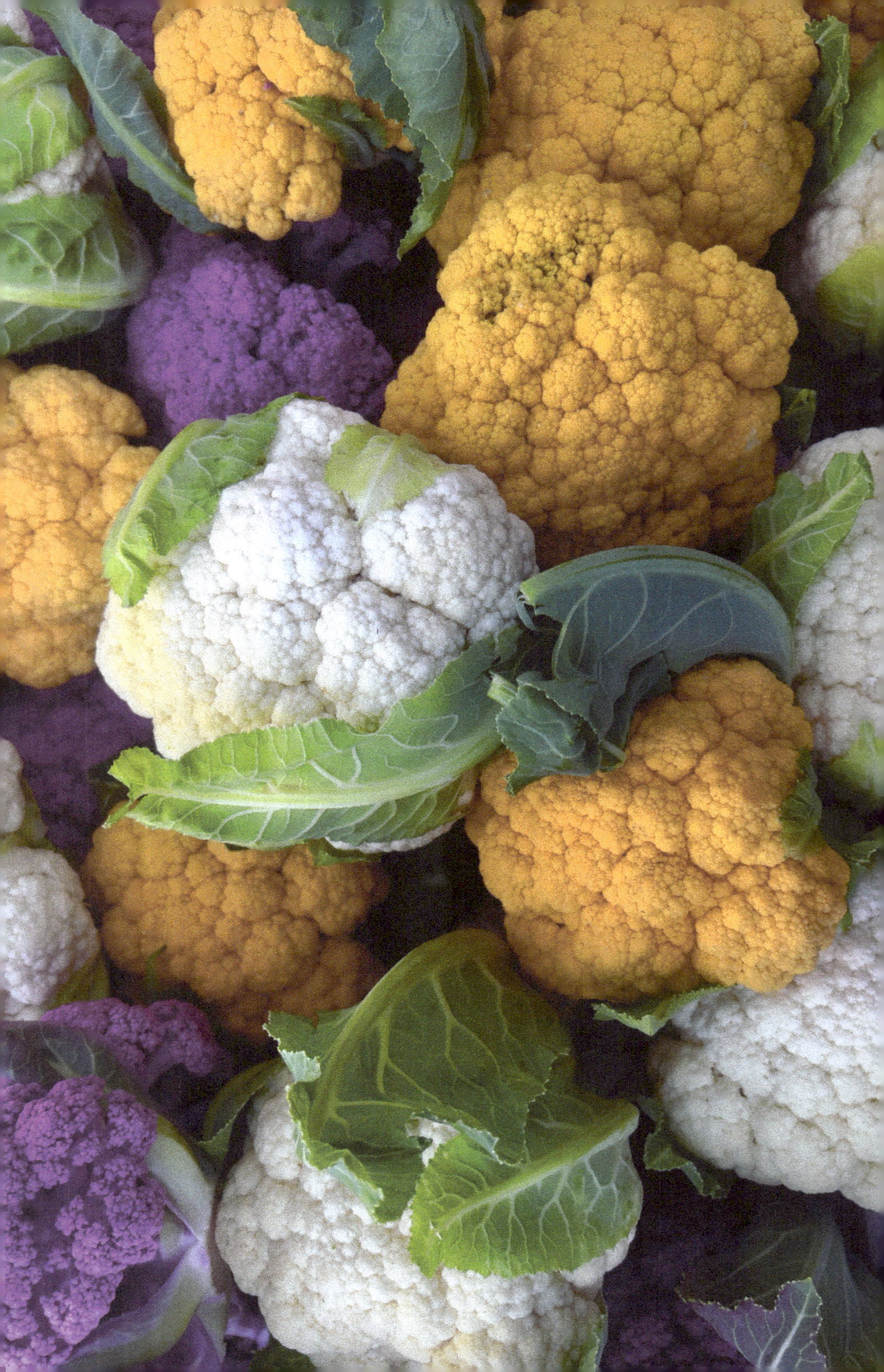

Meatballs and Dairy-Free Cauli Mash

Servings: 3–5 | Prep Time: 10 minutes | Cook Time: 20 minutes

Here we have another dish that offers an alternative option higher in nutrients, by swapping potatoes for cauliflower. While potatoes are not unhealthy, often when they are mashed, it is common to use heavy cream and butter to achieve a creamy texture. The cauliflower provides a low-carb and low-fat option. It also contains fiber, potassium, and vitamins C, K which help your immune system and bone health. The high protein of the meat of your choice also helps repair muscle tissue and will leave you feeling satiated.

This recipe is also provided for this book courtesy of Registered Dietitian Nutritionist Ilana Muhlstein, author of *Love the Food That Loves You Back*. You can find out more about her work by booking a private session with her, purchasing her cookbook, and following her on social media at @ilanamuhlsteinrd.

INGREDIENTS

- 1 pound lean ground beef, turkey, chicken, or vegan alternative
- ⅓ cup almond, coconut, or oat flour
- ¼ cup beef or chicken stock
- 1 tsp avocado or olive oil
- ½ yellow onion, finely chopped
- 1 cup fresh mushrooms, chopped
- 2 cloves garlic, chopped
- 1 egg
- ¼ cup fresh parsley, chopped
- 1 tsp dried basil
- 1 tsp dried oregano
- 1 tsp Worcestershire sauce
- ½ tsp salt, divided
- ½ tsp pepper, divided
- 1 large head or 2 small heads of cauliflower
- ½ cup coconut milk
- ½ tsp dried thyme
- ½ tsp garlic powder
- Salt and pepper to taste for cauli mash

DIRECTIONS

1. Preheat the oven to 400 degrees F. Line a large baking sheet with parchment paper and spray with oil spray.
2. Fill a large pot with water and bring to a boil. Add the whole head of cauliflower or cut up florets and cook until fork tender, about 6 to 8 minutes.
3. In a large bowl, combine the flour and stock and whisk together with a fork or spatula until well combined.

4. Heat a skillet over medium heat. Add the olive oil, mushrooms, and onions and cook down for 2 to 3 minutes. Add in garlic and cook until fragrant. Season with half the salt and pepper.
5. Meanwhile add the meat, egg, Worcestershire, seasonings, herbs, and remaining salt and pepper to the flour and stock mixture.
6. Add the cooked vegetables to the meat mixture and mix well to combine.
7. To streamline the process of forming the balls, form a square with the meat mixture on a baking sheet. If you like bigger meatballs, score four lines across and three lines down, creating twelve even portions of meat; shape them into meatballs.
8. If you prefer smaller meatballs, score four rows by four columns to make 16 evenly sized meatballs, and then shape each portion.
9. Cook for 18 to 22 minutes or until fully cooked through. Exact cooking time will vary based on the size of your meatballs.
10. To make the cauli mash: Strain the cauliflower and add to a food processor or blender with coconut milk, thyme, and garlic powder.
11. Add more coconut milk if needed to reach desired consistency.
12. Add salt and pepper to taste. Serve 2 to 3 cups (250 to 375 grams) of cauli mash along with your meatballs, garnish with parsley and lemon (optional), and enjoy.

Nutritional Facts (per serving):	
Disclaimer: *Nutritional values are estimates and may vary by ingredients and preparation.*	
Serves	4
Serving Size	~3 meatballs + ¾ cup cauliflower mash (~300–350 g total)
Calories	~330 kcal
Protein	23 g
Carbohydrates	12 g
Fiber	4 g
Sugars	3 g (from cauliflower and onions)
Fats	20 g
Saturated Fat	6 g
Unsaturated Fat	14 g
Sodium	~480 mg
Vitamin A	~8% DV
Vitamin C	~90% DV
Calcium	~6% DV
Iron	~20% DV
Magnesium	~15% DV
Potassium	~700 mg
Antioxidants	High (from herbs, garlic, mushrooms, cauliflower, and onion)

Kale Pesto Pasta

Serves: 4–6 | *Prep Time: 5 minutes* | *Cook Time: 20 minutes*

In this recipe, you can choose whichever pasta you prefer, however, it might be helpful to know there are some options on the market with additional benefits aside from the high carbohydrate content. For example, pasta made from lentils or peas with high protein and fiber could be a good choice for this recipe as well. Whether you are carb loading or not, any pasta will do, because the star of this recipe is the kale which has many beneficial nutrients.

INGREDIENTS

Pesto

- 3 cups kale
- 1 garlic clove
- Juice of ½ a lemon
- ½ cup olive oil, plus more for cooking
- ½ cup pine nuts (or sub pumpkin seeds)
- ½ cup freshly grated Parmesan cheese (and more for topping)
- ¼ cup parsley

Pasta

- 4 cups of pasta of choice
- 1 lb chicken breast
- 1 zucchini, thinly sliced
- 1.5 cups grape tomatoes, halved
- Fresh basil leaves for topping

DIRECTIONS

1. Add all ingredients for pesto and blend in a food processor or traditional blender. Adjust salt and pepper to taste. If too dry, add a bit more olive oil. If too wet, sprinkle in more nuts, Parmesan, and kale.
2. Chop your chicken breast into bite-sized pieces. Heat up some olive oil in a pan and cook over medium heat for about 10 minutes.
3. While your chicken is going, slice your tomatoes and zucchini.
4. Add and allow it to cook for another 10 minutes.
5. Boil the water for your pasta and add about 1 Tbsp of salt to it. Once boiling, add your pasta and cook according to package directions.

6. Once pasta is finished, drain it. Combine the pesto and chicken-veggie mixture. Top with basil and enjoy.

Nutritional Facts (per serving):	
Disclaimer: *Nutritional values are estimates and may vary by ingredients and preparation.*	
Serves	**4-6**
Serving Size	**~1¼–1½ cups (~350–400 g)**
Calories	**~490 kcal**
Protein	**27 g**
Carbohydrates	**32 g**
Fiber	**4 g**
Sugars	**4 g (from tomatoes and zucchini)**
Fats	**29 g**
Saturated Fat	**5 g**
Unsaturated Fat	**24 g**
Sodium	**~390 mg**
Vitamin A	**~40% DV**
Vitamin C	**~50% DV**
Calcium	**~20% DV**
Iron	**~15% DV**
Magnesium	**~18% DV**
Potassium	**~650 mg**
Antioxidants	**High (from kale, parsley, garlic, basil, and vegetables)**

Mediterranean Style Fish

Serves: 2 | Cook time: 20 minutes

This is a simple traditional dish you might find in a home or restaurant anywhere from Italy to Greece. Like many Mediterranean dishes, this one is simple but tasty and healthy. Countries in this part of the world tend to use fresher ingredients with an emphasis on healthy fats and lean proteins. You can whip up this nutritious recipe quickly with no need to be an expert in the kitchen, as the most challenging part is chopping tomatoes! You should keep an eye on it and check the fish isn't getting stuck to the pan every few minutes, but mostly you can let the fish do its thing.

INGREDIENTS

- Olive oil to cook
- 2 cloves garlic, whole
- 2 filets white fish of choice
- 2 cups grape tomatoes,
- Black olives of choice, about 10
- 3 cups spinach
- Spices: 3 sprigs of thyme, salt and pepper to taste
- Rice of choice

DIRECTIONS

1. Warm the olive oil in a large flat pan, enough to coat the entire bottom.
2. Once warm, add the garlic, fish, and spices (shred 2 sprigs of thyme and sprinkle over both fish, the other 1 spring you can add whole into the cooking oil).
3. Let simmer on low-medium heat for 10 minutes. While you are waiting, slice the tomatoes and olives in halves.
4. Carefully flip the fish over and add the tomatoes, adding more olive oil if needed.
5. Simmer for another 10 minutes. Then, add the olives and spinach and combine with the now-soft tomatoes.
6. For additional Mediterranean flare, you can also serve it with the Colorful Greek Salad (page 220) or with your choice of rice as a side.

Nutritional Facts (per serving):	
Disclaimer: *Nutritional values are estimates and may vary by ingredients and preparation.*	
Serves	2
Serving Size	1 filet with veggies (~300–350 g)
Calories	~280 kcal
Protein	28 g
Carbohydrates	6 g
Fiber	2.5 g
Sugars	3 g (naturally from tomatoes)
Fats	14 g
Saturated Fat	2 g
Unsaturated Fat	12 g
Sodium	~400 mg (from olives and added salt)
Vitamin A	~70% DV
Vitamin C	~40% DV
Calcium	~8% DV
Iron	~10% DV
Magnesium	~12% DV
Potassium	~650 mg
Antioxidants	High (from tomatoes, spinach, garlic, and olives)

Kale Quinoa Fall Bowl

Serves: 2–4 | *Prep Time: 5 minutes* | *Cook Time: 45 minutes*

Bowls are one of my favorite meals, as you can add a variety of ingredients to give more taste and nutrients. Creating a fall bowl does not always have to be in the autumn, as these ingredients are usually available year-round. If there is an ingredient that you can't locate, however, feel free to substitute it for the next best thing (for example, spinach instead of kale, or raw apple slices instead of pomegranate seeds). In this bowl, you not only have anti-inflammatory fruits and veggies, you also have great macros with protein and carbs. As you will see, I left the protein choice up to you. However, I will offer some recommendations if needed: Turmeric Roasted Chickpeas (page 266), Perla's Perfect Salmon (page 170), grilled chicken breast, or a couple of boiled eggs. If you would like to meal prep this salad you can easily do so. I would simply advise you to wait to massage the kale until you are ready to eat it, so it does not wilt.

INGREDIENTS

- 2 large sweet potatoes
- 2 cups cooked quinoa
- ½ cup pumpkin seeds
- Bunch of kale of choice
- Olive oil for dressing
- ½ cup lemon juice, separated
- 1 small red onion, thinly sliced
- 4 Tbsp of pomegranate seeds
- Protein of choice
- 1 Tbsp maple syrup
- ¼ cup tahini
- 1 tsp garlic powder
- Salt and pepper to taste

DIRECTIONS

1. Prepare a baking sheet and preheat your oven to 350 F. Wash and chop your sweet potatoes into small, bite-sized pieces, season with desired spices, and bake for 30–40 minutes.
2. In the meanwhile, cook your quinoa and protein (see box description for suggestions). Set aside and keep warm.
3. In a flat pan, lightly toast your pumpkin seeds for about 3–5 minutes. Make sure to keep an eye on them as they burn easily.
4. Wash, dry, and thinly slice your kale. Massage it in a bowl with olive oil, ¼ lemon juice, salt, and pepper.

5. Assemble the salad dressing by combining the other ¼ lemon juice, olive oil, maple syrup, garlic powder, and tahini.
6. Once all ingredients are cooked, assemble the bowl starting with the kale. Add desired portions of quinoa, protein, sweet potato, onion, and seeds on top. Lastly, add dressing, combine it all together, and enjoy!

Nutritional Facts (per serving):	
Disclaimer: *Nutritional values are estimates and may vary by ingredients and preparation.*	
Serves	4
Serving Size	~1 bowl (~400–450 g)
Calories	~480 kcal
Protein	20 g
Carbohydrates	42 g
Fiber	7 g
Sugars	6 g (from sweet potatoes, maple syrup, and pomegranate)
Fats	26 g
Saturated Fat	3.5 g
Unsaturated Fat	22.5 g
Sodium	~280 mg (varies based on salt used)
Vitamin A	~180% DV
Vitamin C	~70% DV
Calcium	~15% DV
Iron	~25% DV
Magnesium	~30% DV
Potassium	~750 mg
Antioxidants	Very high (from kale, pomegranate seeds, sweet potatoes, tahini, and lemon)

Turmeric Butternut Squash Soup

Prep Time: 5 minutes | *Cook Time: 30 minutes* | *Serves: 4–6*

Soups are a favorite dish of mine. You can pack many nutrients in them, and they offer a warm and comforting meal. You can also prepare a big batch for the week, or freeze it inside an ice cube tray (broken up into cubes, you are able to control the portion you want to defrost). This recipe is anti-inflammatory and filled with many different veggies, therefore it's an excellent option for your healing journey. If butternut squash is not available, you can use three sweet potatoes instead. For the broth, you can soak bouillon cubes inside simmering water.

INGREDIENTS

- 1 large butternut squash
- 3 large carrots
- 1 medium red onion
- 2 cups broccoli
- 1 red pepper
- 3 cloves of garlic
- 2 tsp of ground turmeric or 3 inches fresh
- 4–6 cups of broth
- 1 can of coconut milk
- 2–3 sprigs of parsley
- Olive oil
- Salt and pepper to taste

DIRECTIONS

1. Prepare a baking sheet with parchment paper and preheat your oven to 325 degrees F.
2. Cut up all your veggies and season with olive oil, salt, pepper, and your preferred spices.
3. Spread out veggies on a baking sheet and bake for 30 minutes or until well roasted (check butternut squash with a fork).
4. Once done, add your roasted veggies, broth, and coconut milk to a blender and blend until smooth. Serve with some additional parsley as garnish.

Nutritional Facts (per serving):	
Disclaimer: *Nutritional values are estimates and may vary by ingredients and preparation.*	
Serves	6
Serving Size	~1½ cups (~350–400 g)
Calories	~210 kcal
Protein	3 g
Carbohydrates	23 g
Fiber	5 g
Sugars	8 g (naturally from vegetables)
Fats	13 g
Saturated Fat	10 g
Unsaturated Fat	3 g
Sodium	~380 mg (based on broth and added salt)
Vitamin A	~280% DV
Vitamin C	~90% DV
Calcium	~8% DV
Iron	~15% DV
Magnesium	~14% DV
Potassium	~600 mg
Antioxidants	Very high (from turmeric, parsley, garlic, and colorful vegetables)

Enchilada Quinoa Bake

Servings: 2–4 | *Cook Time: 1 hour*

When you are craving Mexican inspired cuisine that will leave you full and satisfied, this is a great dish to try. This recipe is full of protein and fiber, essential for healing and keeping your digestion normal. While it takes about an hour to cook, the majority of it is simply waiting for the oven to do its thing. Like many of the dishes in this book, you can double it and save some for later in the week.

This dish is provided courtesy of Dini Klein, the creator of Prep + Rally (prepandrally.com) where Dini shares kid-friendly clean meals. Dini is a food host, former private chef, wife, and loving parent, so she knows what it is like to be busy with very little time to cook. However, she also knows how important it is to eat nutritious and wholesome meals. You can find more satisfying meal inspiration by following Dini at @prepandrally on all socials.

INGREDIENTS

- 3 cups dry quinoa
- 5.25 cups vegetable broth
- 2 cups sautéed peppers and onions
- 1 15 ounce cans black beans, drained and rinsed
- 1 15 ounce can fire roasted diced tomatoes
- 1 cup red enchilada sauce
- 1 1 ounce packet taco seasoning
- 2 15 oz cans corn kernels, drained
- 1 cup shredded mozzarella or cheddar for topping

DIRECTIONS

1. Preheat the oven to 400 degrees.
2. Add the quinoa and vegetable broth to a saucepan and bring to a boil. Cover and reduce the heat to low.
3. Cook covered for 15–20 minutes or until the liquid is gone. Remove from the heat and let sit for 10 minutes. Fluff with a fork.
4. Reserve 3 cups for the enchilada bake and store the rest for another time, such as for the Anti-Inflammatory BBQ Chicken Quinoa Bowl (page 199) or Build Your Own Buddha Bowl (page 206).
5. In a large bowl, mix together 3 cups of cooked quinoa with the remaining ingredients (besides the shredded cheese) until fully combined. Pour into an oven-safe baking dish and top with cheese.

6. Bake for about 30-40 minutes or until the edges are bubbly and the cheese is melted. Serve with desired garnishes and enjoy!

Nutritional Facts (per serving):	
Disclaimer: *Nutritional values are estimates and may vary by ingredients and preparation.*	
Serves	**4**
Serving Size	**~2 cups (~450–500 g)**
Calories	**~550 kcal**
Protein	**21 g**
Carbohydrates	**66 g**
Fiber	**10 g**
Sugars	**9 g (from corn, tomatoes, peppers, onions)**
Fats	**22 g**
Saturated Fat	**7 g**
Unsaturated Fat	**15 g**
Sodium	**~900 mg (from broth, canned goods, seasoning)**
Vitamin A	**~20% DV**
Vitamin C	**~50% DV**
Calcium	**~30% DV**
Iron	**~30% DV**
Magnesium	**~35% DV**
Potassium	**~950 mg**
Antioxidants	**High (from quinoa, beans, tomatoes, peppers, onions, and spices)**

Salmon with Tahini Yogurt Sauce

Servings: 4 **|** *Cook Time: 15 minutes*

While you can't go wrong with any type of salmon, this dish by Prep + Rally offers a fresh Greek-inspired twist. Tzatziki sauce is a light and fresh addition to it, and I have tried it so often that I can make it without the recipe now. You can pair this dish with a side carb of your choice, such as asparagus, potatoes, basmati rice, etc. There is really no way to go wrong. With the micro and macronutrient-rich salmon, any addition adds extra goodness to this already healthy dish. Once you give this a try, I am certain it will become a favorite of yours as well.

This dish is also provided courtesy of Dini Klein, the foodie and creator of Prep + Rally (prepandrally.com). Even if you are busy, Dini will help you stick to your goals for a healthy eating lifestyle by offering vibrant and simple meal options. You can find more of her meals by following Dini at @prepandrally on all socials.

INGREDIENTS

- 2 cups plain Greek yogurt
- ¼ cup tahini
- 2 Tbsp fresh dill, minced
- 2 Tbsp fresh mint,minced
- 1 lemon, juiced
- 2 cloves garlic, minced
- Salt and pepper to season
- 4 6–8 oz salmon filets

DIRECTIONS

1. Add all sauce ingredients to a medium bowl and whisk to combine.
2. Heat the grill to medium high heat, about 450 degrees. Lightly oil the salmon filets and season with a pinch of salt and pepper.
3. When the grill is hot, place the salmon skin side up on the grill. Grill for 3-6 minutes per side, depending on the thickness of the salmon, until cooked through. Remove from the heat.
4. Serve the salmon with the tahini yogurt sauce on top or underneath.

Nutritional Facts (per serving):	
Disclaimer: *Nutritional values are estimates and may vary by ingredients and preparation.*	
Serves	4
Serving Size	1 salmon filet (~6–8 oz) + ~¼ cup sauce (~250–300 g total)
Calories	~450 kcal
Protein	40 g
Carbohydrates	4 g
Fiber	1 g
Sugars	2 g (naturally from yogurt and lemon)
Fats	30 g
Saturated Fat	6 g
Unsaturated Fat	24 g
Sodium	~280 mg
Vitamin A	~6% DV
Vitamin C	~10% DV
Calcium	~15% DV
Iron	~10% DV
Magnesium	~15% DV
Potassium	~850 mg
Antioxidants	Moderate to high (from herbs, garlic, lemon, and tahini)

Greek Yogurt Lemon Chicken Thighs

Servings: 3 **|** *Prep Time: 5 minutes* **|** *Cook Time: 30 minutes*

If you are looking for a high protein dish but are tired of fish or plain chicken breast, give yourself a break and go for these yummy chicken thighs. While thighs are slightly higher in fat, they are still high in protein and offer a moist and delicious alternative to indulge in every once in a while. By adding the Greek yogurt to this recipe, you have an excellent high protein option that can be made with very little effort.

INGREDIENTS

- 6 bone-in, skin-on chicken thighs
- ¾ cup Greek yogurt
- Juice of ½ lemon
- 1 Tbsp olive oil
- 1 tsp of salt, pepper, garlic powder

DIRECTIONS

1. In a bowl, combine Greek yogurt, lemon juice, olive oil, and seasonings.
2. Add chicken thighs and mix until fully coated.
3. Cover and marinate in the fridge for at least 1 hour, preferably overnight.
4. Preheat the air fryer to 350 degrees F. Add chicken thighs in a single layer.
5. Cook at 350 degrees F for 15–18 minutes.
6. Increase heat to 400 degrees F and cook for another 5–7 minutes to crisp the skin and brown the edges.
7. Take out and let rest 3–5 minutes before serving.

Nutritional Facts (per serving):	
Disclaimer: *Nutritional values are estimates and may vary by ingredients and preparation.*	
Serves	3
Serving Size	2 chicken thighs (~175–200 g cooked)
Calories	~320 kcal
Protein	32 g
Carbohydrates	2 g
Fiber	0 g
Sugars	1 g (from yogurt and lemon juice)
Fats	20 g
Saturated Fat	6 g
Unsaturated Fat	14 g
Sodium	~550 mg (varies depending on added salt)
Vitamin A	~2% DV
Vitamin C	~6% DV
Calcium	~6% DV
Iron	~10% DV
Magnesium	~8% DV
Potassium	~300 mg
Antioxidants	Moderate (from garlic powder and lemon)

NOTES

If you don't have an air fryer, roast the thighs in the oven for 30–40 minutes at 400 degrees F, checking every so often.

Low Carb Cheesy Tuna Patty

Servings: 2 patties | *Prep Time: 5 minutes* | *Cook Time: 10 minutes*

As we have uncovered earlier in the book, protein is an essential building block to healing. Integrating protein into every meal is the easiest way to make sure you are getting the quantity you need. This delicious dish creates a high protein burger that you will want on repeat. As it is low carb, you can also eat this if following a keto diet or simply want to be conscious of your carb intake. I advise doubling or tripling the amount into order to freeze some for later.

INGREDIENTS

- 1 (5-ounce) can tuna packed in water, drained
- 1 large egg, whisked
- ¼ cup shredded cheddar cheese (about 1 ounce)
- Pinch of kosher salt
- 1 Tbsp salted butter, for the pan

DIRECTIONS

1. Put the tuna, egg, and cheese in a medium-size bowl. Season with the salt and mix well with a fork to combine the ingredients.
2. Divide the tuna mixture into 2 equal portions and shape each portion into a patty about ½-inch thick.
3. Preheat a large skillet over medium-high heat until hot but not yet smoking, about 3 minutes.
4. Drop in the butter and swirl to coat the pan. Place the patties in the pan and pan-fry for 2 to 3 minutes, until browned on the bottom. Flip and cook for 2 to 3 minutes more, until browned on the other side.
5. Serve immediately with a knife and fork, or let cool for a few minutes until easy to handle and eat as a handheld meal.

Nutritional Facts (per serving):	
Disclaimer: *Nutritional values are estimates and may vary by ingredients and preparation.*	
Serves	1
Serving Size	Entire recipe (~160–180 g cooked)
Calories	~330 kcal
Protein	32 g
Carbohydrates	1 g
Fiber	0 g
Sugars	0 g
Fats	22 g
Saturated Fat	11 g
Unsaturated Fat	11 g
Sodium	~600 mg (from tuna, cheese, butter, and salt)
Vitamin A	~10% DV
Vitamin C	~0% DV
Calcium	~20% DV
Iron	~10% DV
Magnesium	~6% DV
Potassium	~250 mg
Antioxidants	Moderate (mainly from egg yolk and cheddar)

Sweet & Salty Harvest Bowl

Servings: 1–2 | Prep Time: 10 minutes | Cook Time: 30 minutes

This bowl offers an excellent range of macro and micronutrients. With the complex carbs of the sweet potato and rice, the lean proteins you choose, the healthy fats via the avocado and tahini, and the kale, you get a wonderful rainbow of nutrients in this dish. I personally love sweet and salty dishes, so this one is on repeat in my home!

INGREDIENTS

Bowl Base

- 1 sweet potato
- ½ cup wild rice
- ½ cup roasted pecans (sautéed in a little butter)
- 4 cups sautéed kale
- ½ avocado
- ¼ cup raisins
- Protein of choice (optional)

Turmeric Tahini Dressing

- ½ cup tahini
- 1 tsp turmeric
- 1–2 garlic cloves
- 1 Tbsp olive oil
- 1 Tbsp maple syrup
- Lemon juice
- Black pepper
- Sea Salt
- ⅛–¼ cup water

DIRECTIONS

1. Prepare a baking sheet and preheat your oven to 400 degrees F. Cube the sweet potato, coat with olive oil, salt, and pepper. Roast for about 30 minutes.
2. While that is cooking, prepare your rice, roast your pecans with a bit of butter, and sauté your kale. Slice your avocado and set out the portion of raisins.
3. Next, blend all the ingredients for the tahini dressing.
4. Once all ingredients are ready, assemble, drizzle with dressing, and enjoy!

Nutritional Facts (per serving):	
Disclaimer: *Nutritional values are estimates and may vary by ingredients and preparation.*	
Serves	2
Serving Size	~1 bowl (~450–500 g)
Calories	~620 kcal
Protein	12 g
Carbohydrates	48 g
Fiber	10 g
Sugars	10 g (from sweet potato, raisins, and maple syrup)
Fats	42 g
Saturated Fat	6 g
Unsaturated Fat	36 g
Sodium	~250 mg (depends on salt added to dressing)
Vitamin A	~300% DV
Vitamin C	~70% DV
Calcium	~15% DV
Iron	~25% DV
Magnesium	~35% DV
Potassium	~900 mg
Antioxidants	Very high (from turmeric, kale, sweet potato, garlic, and raisins)

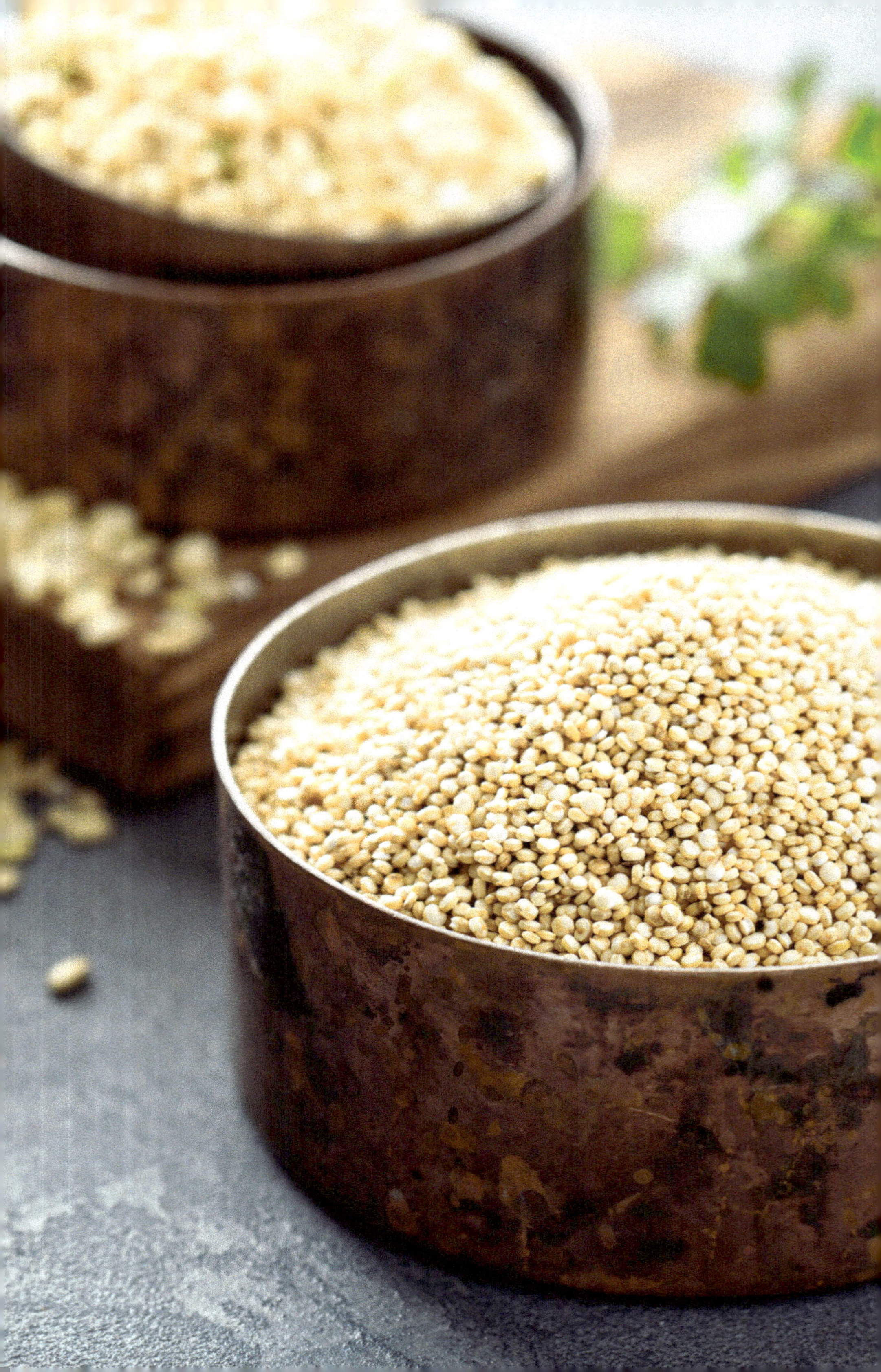

Anti-Inflammatory BBQ Chicken Quinoa Bowl

Servings: 4 | *Cook Time: 30 minutes*

Cooking on a barbeque is a very nostalgic activity because it makes me remember fun family celebrations and national holidays, and the flavor of BBQ sauce brings a similar feeling. This is a healthy and fresh dish that has a lot of flavor and is packed with both macro and micronutrients. While you can technically put BBQ sauce on anything, the flavors included in this dish combine nicely to create something special.

INGREDIENTS

Base

- 1 cup quinoa

Veggies

- 2 sweet potatoes, diced in cubes and roasted
- 5–6 mini bell peppers
- 2 cups cherry tomatoes
- 1 red onion, sliced
- 2 jalapeños
- 1 Tbsp olive oil
- 2 tsp salt
- 2 tsp paprika
- 1 tsp chili powder
- 1 tsp cumin
- Black pepper

Chicken

- 2 chicken breasts, cubed
- Salt & pepper
- 1 cup plain Greek yogurt
- ¼ tsp chili flakes
- 2 tsp paprika
- 2 tsp chili powder
- 2 tsp cumin
- 1 tsp cayenne
- 1 tsp garlic powder
- 1 tsp onion powder
- 2 limes, juiced
- 1 Tbsp honey

Creamy BBQ Sauce

- ½ cup Greek yogurt or sour cream
- ½ cup BBQ sauce
- 1 tsp chili powder

Toppings

- ½ cup aged cheddar (divided)
- 1 handful cilantro (optional)
- Black pepper
- 1 avocado, thinly sliced

DIRECTIONS

1. Preheat your oven to 400 degrees and prepare 2 baking sheets. Cube your sweet potatoes and cook on the first baking sheet for about 30 minutes.
2. On the second sheet, toss remaining veggies in the spices and olive oil and roast in the oven as well for about 20 minutes.
3. While those two things are cooking, prepare your quinoa.
4. Mix the "Chicken" ingredients together in a bowl and coat your chicken with it. Cook your chicken in a pan on the stovetop.
5. Last but not least, mix your Cream BBQ Sauce and set aside. Optionally, you can put it in a Ziploc bag in order to properly drizzle it on top.
6. Assemble all the ingredients together once ready, drizzle with your sauce, and enjoy!

Nutritional Facts (per serving):	
Disclaimer: *Nutritional values are estimates and may vary by ingredients and preparation.*	
Serves	4
Serving Size	~1 loaded bowl (~500–550 g)
Calories	~580 kcal
Protein	38 g
Carbohydrates	36 g
Fiber	7 g
Sugars	10 g (from sweet potatoes, BBQ sauce, and veggies)
Fats	30 g
Saturated Fat	8 g
Unsaturated Fat	22 g
Sodium	~600 mg
Vitamin A	~120% DV
Vitamin C	~90% DV
Calcium	~20% DV
Iron	~20% DV
Magnesium	~25% DV
Potassium	~900 mg
Antioxidants	Very high (from peppers, spices, avocado, lime, and sweet potato)

Creamy Vegetable Soup

Servings: 4–6 **|** *Prep Time: 10 minutes* **|** *Cook Time: 45 minutes*

Creamy soups have a special place in my heart because they remind me of rainy days. I usually like to eat them with a warm toasted slice of bread as well, which somehow feels nostalgic. My opinion on this one is that the combination of the herbs, coconut, and vegetables creates a fragrant yet classic flavor. Like most soups, while the cooking time is about forty minutes, most of that time you are just letting the veggies do their thing while you relax.

INGREDIENTS

- 6 Roma tomatoes, halved
- 4 carrots, peeled and halved
- 1 red pepper, cut into quarters
- 1 white onion, halved
- 2 garlic bulbs
- 2 zucchinis, sliced
- 2 Tbsp olive oil
- Salt and pepper
- 2 tsp dried basil
- 1 tsp Italian seasonings
- 1 tsp dried oregano
- 2½ cups water, boiled
- 1 cup milk or coconut milk
- Handful fresh basil

DIRECTIONS

1. Preheat the oven to 425 degrees F. Line the baking sheet with parchment paper and set aside.
2. Wash and chop all veggies. Add to a lined baking sheet and toss with olive oil and seasonings until evenly coated.
3. Add garlic to tin foil, season and wrap and place on the lined baking sheet. Cook for 40-45 minutes. Check on veggies half way.
4. Once veggies are cooked, add all veggies to a food processor or blender. Squeeze in roasted garlic once cooled. Add in salt and pepper, and boiling water. Blend until smooth. Add in milk and blend. If you want your soup thinner—add more water as needed.
5. Add soup to bowls and add milk, black pepper and fresh basil on top. If your soup needs to be at a warmer temperature—add to a large pot and bring to a boil. Serve with toasted bread and enjoy!

Nutritional Facts (per serving):	
Disclaimer: *Nutritional values are estimates and may vary by ingredients and preparation.*	
Serves	4
Serving Size	~1½–2 cups (~400–450 g)
Calories	~180 kcal
Protein	4 g
Carbohydrates	20 g
Fiber	6 g
Sugars	10 g (naturally from carrots, tomatoes, and onions)
Fats	10 g
Saturated Fat	5 g
Unsaturated Fat	5 g
Sodium	~280 mg (depends on added salt and broth)
Vitamin A	~160% DV
Vitamin C	~100% DV
Calcium	~8% DV
Iron	~10% DV
Magnesium	~12% DV
Potassium	~850 mg
Antioxidants	Very high (from tomatoes, garlic, carrots, basil, zucchini, and red pepper)

Creamy Chicken Piccata

Servings: 2–4 | *Prep Time: 5 minutes* | *Cook Time: 20 minutes*

The dish Chicken Piccata traditionally is made with normal flour which contains gluten and lots of butter and cream. This variation calls for gluten-free flour to avoid any inflammatory response and coconut cream instead of regular cream, as the latter contains more saturated fat. If you are not a coconut fan, in my opinion, the taste of the coconut with the lemon and herbs disguises the sweetness of the coconut and creates a delicious savory taste.

INGREDIENTS

- 1½ lbs boneless, skinless chicken breasts pounded to ½-inch thickness
- Sea salt and freshly ground black pepper
- ¼ cup gluten-free flour
- 3 Tbsp olive oil divided
- 1 small onion chopped
- 4 garlic cloves minced
- 1 cup chicken bone broth
- 1 lemon juiced
- ½ cup coconut cream, blended before using
- ¼ cup capers drained
- Lemon wedges to serve
- Freshly chopped herbs to garnish

DIRECTIONS

1. Season the pounded chicken with a pinch of salt and pepper on both sides. Place the flour in a shallow bowl.
2. Heat 2 Tbsp of the oil in a large skillet over medium heat. Working with one cutlet at a time, dredge the chicken on both sides in the flour. Shake off the excess flour, and add them to the skillet.
3. Cook the chicken for 4 minutes per side, or until the chicken is cooked through and the coating is golden brown. Transfer the browned chicken to a plate, and set aside.
4. In the same pan, lower the heat to medium-low, and add the remaining Tbsp of oil, onions, and garlic. Sauté for 2–3 minutes, stirring occasionally, until the onions are softened.
5. Add the broth and lemon juice, and scrape the browned bits from the bottom of the pan with a silicone spatula. Raise the heat to medium-high, and boil the mixture for 3 minutes, until reduced by half, stirring occasionally.

6. Stir in the coconut cream and capers, and settle the chicken into the sauce. Simmer for 2-3 minutes, over low heat, or unti heated through. Season to taste with sea salt and black pepper.
7. Serve warm over sautéed cauliflower or cooked rice.

Nutritional Facts (per serving):	
Disclaimer: *Nutritional values are estimates and may vary by ingredients and preparation.*	
Serves	**4**
Serving Size	**~1 chicken breast + sauce (~250–300 g)**
Calories	**~360 kcal**
Protein	**35 g**
Carbohydrates	**6 g**
Fiber	**1 g**
Sugars	**1 g (from onions and coconut cream)**
Fats	**20 g**
Saturated Fat	**7 g**
Unsaturated Fat	**13 g**
Sodium	**~420 mg (includes salt, broth, and capers)**
Vitamin A	**~2% DV**
Vitamin C	**~25% DV**
Calcium	**~2% DV**
Iron	**~8% DV**
Magnesium	**~10% DV**
Potassium	**~550 mg**
Antioxidants	**Moderate to high (from garlic, lemon, herbs, and olive oil)**

Build Your Own Buddha Bowl

Servings: 1 | Cook Time: 20 minutes

Some of the best recipes are ones you can customize, and this is in that category. For this one, I recommend you can choose any slow carb grain such as cooked quinoa, brown rice, buckwheat, or freekeh. For the protein you could select something like fish, tofu, tempeh, or beans. A smart strategy is to cook big portions of the ingredients you like and save them in the fridge or freezer to reheat and customize at a moment's notice.

INGREDIENTS

- ½ cup cooked quinoa (or other grain base of choice
- 3 oz grilled chicken (or other protein of choice)
- 1 cup mixed sautéed veggies (e.g., bell pepper, zucchini, broccoli)
- ¼ avocado, 1 Tbsp extra-virgin olive oil, or seeds for topping
- 1 Tbsp of tahini, Traditional Hummus (page 248), or low-sodium tamari
- Juice of ½ lemon

DIRECTIONS

1. Prepare your grains as directed on the package.
2. While that is going, cook your protein and sauté your veggies unless you are eating them raw.
3. Once all is ready, assemble, add your toppings, and enjoy!

Nutritional Facts (per serving):	
Disclaimer: *Nutritional values are estimates and may vary by ingredients and preparation.*	
Serves	1
Serving Size	1 full bowl (~450–500 g)
Calories	~480 kcal
Protein	30 g
Carbohydrates	30 g
Fiber	8 g
Sugars	4 g (from vegetables)
Fats	28 g
Saturated Fat	4 g
Unsaturated Fat	24 g
Sodium	~220 mg (depends on dressing/salt)
Vitamin A	~60% DV
Vitamin C	~70% DV
Calcium	~10% DV
Iron	~20% DV
Magnesium	~20% DV
Potassium	~750 mg
Antioxidants	High (from colorful veggies, tahini, lemon, and olive oil)

Garlic Butter Baked Salmon

Servings: 4 **|** *Prep Time: 5 minutes* **|** *Cook Time: 15 minutes*

This recipe has a secret ingredient: honey. In my experience, I have never had a bad dish with honey in it. However, sweet and savory dishes might be slightly difficult to get right. Luckily, this one most certainly hits the spot. The balance of spices, butter, honey, and zesty lemon provides an interesting flavor to liven up your regular salt-and-pepper seasoned salmon. This is a very quick dish that you can pair with any side you desire, from brown rice to salad.

INGREDIENTS

- 4 boneless salmon fillets (6–7 oz per portion)
- 2 Tbsp unsalted butter melted
- 2 cloves minced garlic
- 2 Tbsp honey
- ½ tsp dried parsley (or 2 tsp fresh parsley, finely chopped)
- ¼ tsp salt
- ¼ tsp pepper
- Pinch of paprika
- 1 lemon, quartered

DIRECTIONS

1. Preheat the oven to 400 degrees F. Line a baking tray with foil or a silicon mat.
2. Place the salmon fillets, skin-side-down on the baking tray.
3. In a small bowl, mix together the melted butter, garlic, honey, parsley, salt, pepper and paprika.
4. Pour the mixture over the salmon fillets (don't worry about any of the sauce pooling on the tray).
5. Arrange the lemon wedges on and around the salmon.
6. Place in the oven and bake for 8 minutes.
7. Open the oven and baste the salmon with any of the sauce that has pooled on the tray. Bake for a further 4–7 minutes until the salmon is tender.

Nutritional Facts (per serving):	
Disclaimer: *Nutritional values are estimates and may vary by ingredients and preparation.*	
Serves	4
Serving Size	1 salmon fillet with sauce (~180–200 g/ 6-7 oz portion)
Calories	~360 kcal
Protein	34 g
Carbohydrates	6 g
Fiber	0 g
Sugars	5 g (from honey)
Fats	22 g
Saturated Fat	7 g
Unsaturated Fat	15 g
Sodium	~260 mg
Vitamin A	~6% DV
Vitamin C	~10% DV (from lemon)
Calcium	~2% DV
Iron	~6% DV
Magnesium	~10% DV
Potassium	~700 mg
Antioxidants	Moderate (from garlic, parsley, paprika, and lemon)

Tofu Veggie Bowl

Servings: 4 | Prep Time: 10 minutes | Cook Time: 30 minutes

It is always best to try everything in moderation, and the same goes for eating soy products like tofu. It is rich in protein and low in fat, so makes a great substitution to animal protein, however, since it is technically processed, you should have it only occasionally and try your best to get the majority of your protein intake from whole one-ingredient proteins like beans. With that said, this offers a refreshing low-fat option when you want to try something different.

INGREDIENTS

- 14 oz package of tofu
- Store bought BBQ sauce, to taste
- ½ cup bulgur wheat, or other grain of choice
- 1 avocado
- 2 cups broccoli
- 1 cup tomatoes
- 1–2 grated carrots
- 1 Tbsp vegan mayo (Veganaise is a good option)
- Sliced cucumber
- Green lettuce
- Juice of ¼ lemon

DIRECTIONS

1. Prepare a baking sheet and preheat the oven to 350 degrees F. Cube and bake tofu for about 20 minutes, then pull it out to coat the tofu in the BBQ sauce. Return and bake for another 10 minutes.
2. While the tofu is cooking, prepare your bulgur wheat.
3. Chop your veggies and assemble. Top with some mayo and enjoy!

Nutritional Facts (per serving):	
Disclaimer: *Nutritional values are estimates and may vary by ingredients and preparation.*	
Serves	4
Serving Size	~1 bowl (~400–450 g)
Calories	~410 kcal
Protein	16 g
Carbohydrates	38 g
Fiber	8 g
Sugars	8 g (from BBQ sauce, carrots, and tomatoes)
Fats	22 g
Saturated Fat	3.5 g
Unsaturated Fat	18.5 g
Sodium	~450 mg (varies based on BBQ sauce and mayo)
Vitamin A	~90% DV
Vitamin C	~70% DV
Calcium	~20% DV
Iron	~25% DV
Magnesium	~25% DV
Potassium	~750 mg
Antioxidants	High (from broccoli, carrots, avocado, lemon, and tomatoes)

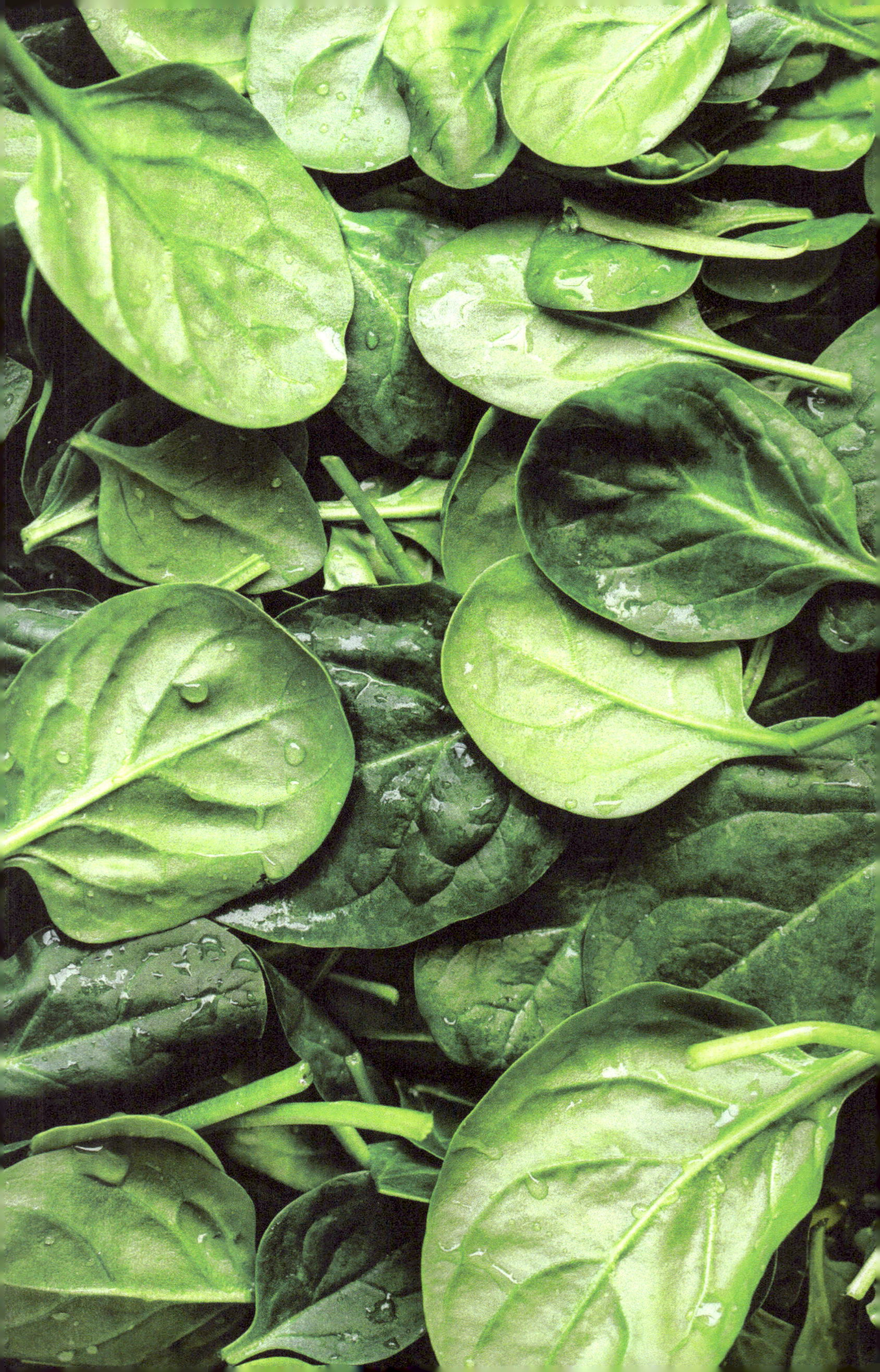

Seared Salmon Over Sautéed Garlic Spinach Tomato

Servings: 2 | Cook Time: 30 minutes

This dish can potentially provide all the key nutrients you need in one meal. As we covered earlier, salmon has high protein and healthy fat. The olives also provide healthy fat. Further, the inclusion of various different vegetables offers ideal micronutrient content. If you would like to add a carb, try some brown rice. However, the dish is also delicious and filling on its own for a lighter meal.

This healthy creation was curated by holistic chef Elizabeth Leigh Mandelbaum. You can purchase her cookbook *Plated* on Amazon which is packed with unique and nutritious recipes. Also, you can discover more of her healthy creations at @elizabethleigh.m on Instagram.

INGREDIENTS

- 2 salmon filets
- 1 shallot
- 4 cloves garlic, crushed
- 8 oz cherry tomatoes
- 8 oz baby bella mushrooms, sliced
- 16 oz fresh spinach
- ½ cup kalamata olives, halved
- ½ tsp onion powder
- ½ tsp paprika
- ½ tsp garlic powder
- Olive oil
- Salt and pepper

DIRECTIONS

For the Salmon

1. Remove the salmon from the refrigerator about 5 minutes before you begin cooking. If you like to rinse your fish, go ahead and rinse the salmon then pat it dry.
2. Sprinkle salt and pepper evenly over the side without skin.
3. Heat a skillet to a medium heat with 1–2 tbsp of the olive oil.
4. Place the salmon skin side down first, even if your salmon is skinless. Let it cook for 3–5 minutes. You will see the color of the fish starting to change from the bottom going upward.

5. When the color has changed half way or even a little bit more, then flip it to the other side. Let the other side cook for another 3–5 minutes. Remove the fish from the pan and repeat the same instructions for the next filet.

For the Garlic Spinach Tomato

1. Heat a skillet with 1–2 tbsp of olive oil. Add the diced shallot, halved cherry tomatoes, crushed garlic and sliced mushrooms to the pan. Saute all together for about 8 minutes, until everything is nice and soft.
2. Then add in the spinach, olives, onion powder, paprika and garlic powder. Stir together until fully combined and cooked.
3. Split the spinach mixture into two, placing each half in the center of a plate. Plate the salmon filets over the bed of spinach. Serve and enjoy!

Nutritional Facts (per serving):	
Disclaimer: *Nutritional values are estimates and may vary by ingredients and preparation.*	
Serves	2
Serving Size	1 salmon filet + sautéed vegetables (~400–450 g)
Calories	~480 kcal
Protein	35 g
Carbohydrates	10 g
Fiber	4 g
Sugars	4 g (from shallots and tomatoes)
Fats	32 g
Saturated Fat	6 g
Unsaturated Fat	26 g
Sodium	~500 mg (from olives and seasoning)
Vitamin A	~120% DV
Vitamin C	~40% DV
Calcium	~8% DV
Iron	~15% DV
Magnesium	~20% DV
Potassium	~950 mg
Antioxidants	Very high (from spinach, tomatoes, garlic, olives, and spices)

NOTES

This recipe can be made with grilled chicken breast or seared boneless steaks as well! To make it vegan, use tofu or vegan meat alternatives in place of the salmon. You can also serve the Garlic Spinach Tomato mixed into a protein based pasta.

Greens Soup

Servings: 4–6 | *Prep Time: 5 minutes* | *Cook Time: 35 minutes*

I never miss an opportunity to pack as many nutrients into one meal as possible, and neither should you. It is the simplest way to make sure you are getting the nutrition you need without needing to take supplements. You can accomplish this with smoothies by disguising kale, cucumber, or spinach among sweeter fruits like pineapple. Or, you can create comforting soups like this.

Similar to the previous recipe, this healthy creation was curated by holistic chef Elizabeth Leigh Mandelbaum who offers clean and vibrant recipes on her platform. You can purchase her cookbook *Plated* on Amazon which is packed with unique and nutritious recipes. Also, you can discover more of her healthy creations at @elizabethleigh.m on Instagram.

INGREDIENTS

- 1 brown onion, diced
- 8–10 cloves garlic, crushed
- 4 large zucchini, cut into fours
- 24 oz frozen broccoli
- ½ cup chopped cilantro
- ½ cup chopped parsley
- 1 tsp onion powder
- 1 tsp garlic powder
- Olive oil
- Salt and pepper

DIRECTIONS

1. Heat a large pot with 1-2 tsp of the olive oil and saute the diced onion, and crushed garlic.
2. Then add the zucchini and frozen broccoli.
3. Cover with water and bring to a boil. Let it boil for 15 minutes then turn the flame to a simmer and cover the pot. Let it cook for about an hour, until the veggies are super soft.
4. Then add the cilantro and parsley and cook for another 20 minutes. Strain the water then add the spices, salt and pepper.
5. Then using an immersion blender, blend the veggies until smooth, leaving no clumps. If you don't have an immersion blender, wait for the veggies to cool, then transfer to a blender and blend well. Serve and enjoy!

Nutritional Facts (per serving):	
Disclaimer: *Nutritional values are estimates and may vary by ingredients and preparation.*	
Serves	**4**
Serving Size	**~1½–2 cups (~350–400 g)**
Calories	**~110 kcal**
Protein	**5 g**
Carbohydrates	**13 g**
Fiber	**5 g**
Sugars	**5 g (naturally from zucchini and onion)**
Fats	**5 g**
Saturated Fat	**0.7 g**
Unsaturated Fat	**4.3 g**
Sodium	**~220 mg (varies based on added salt)**
Vitamin A	**~35% DV**
Vitamin C	**~80% DV**
Calcium	**~8% DV**
Iron	**~10% DV**
Magnesium	**~15% DV**
Potassium	**~700 mg**
Antioxidants	**Very high (from garlic, herbs, broccoli, and zucchini)**

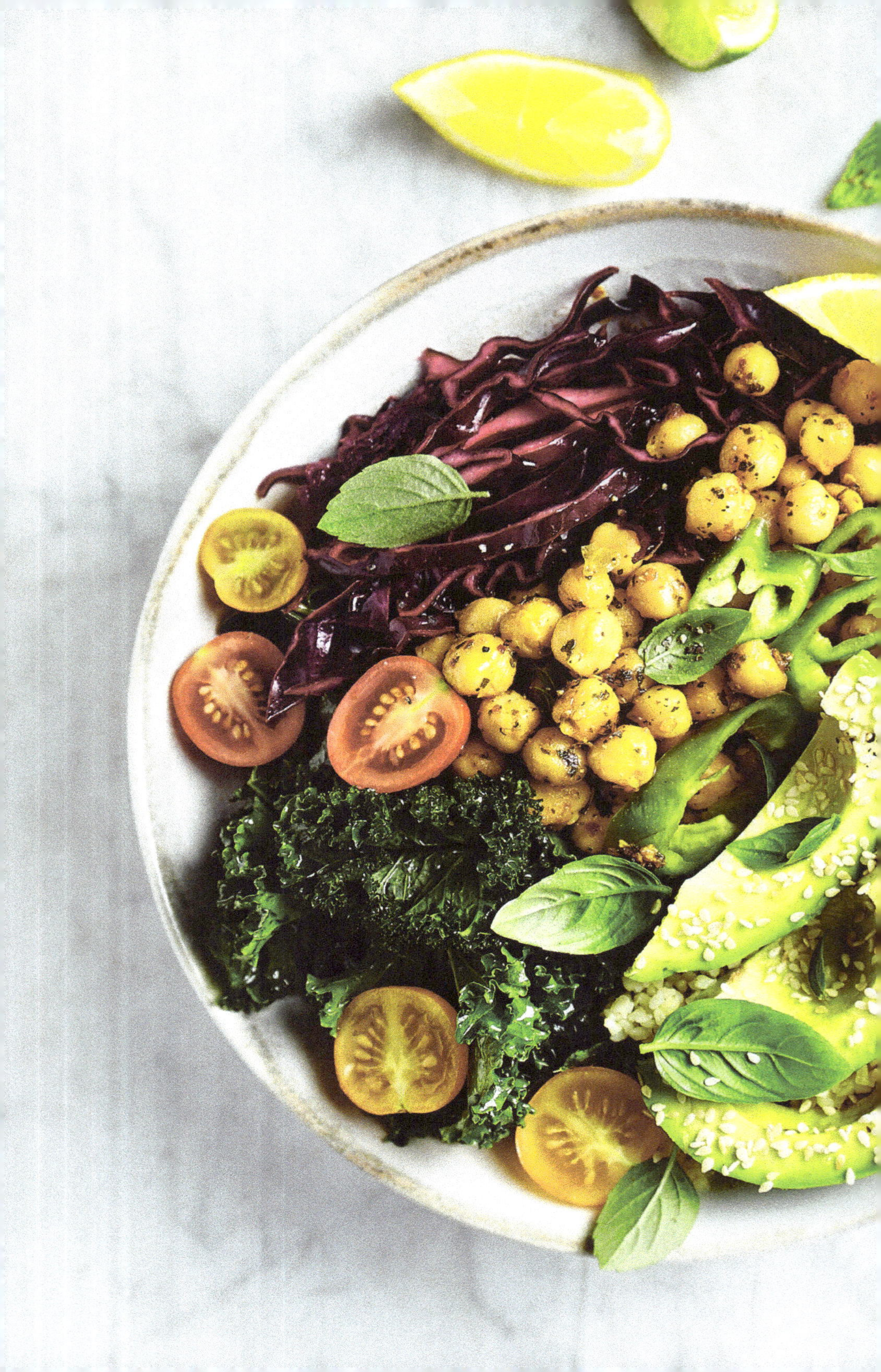

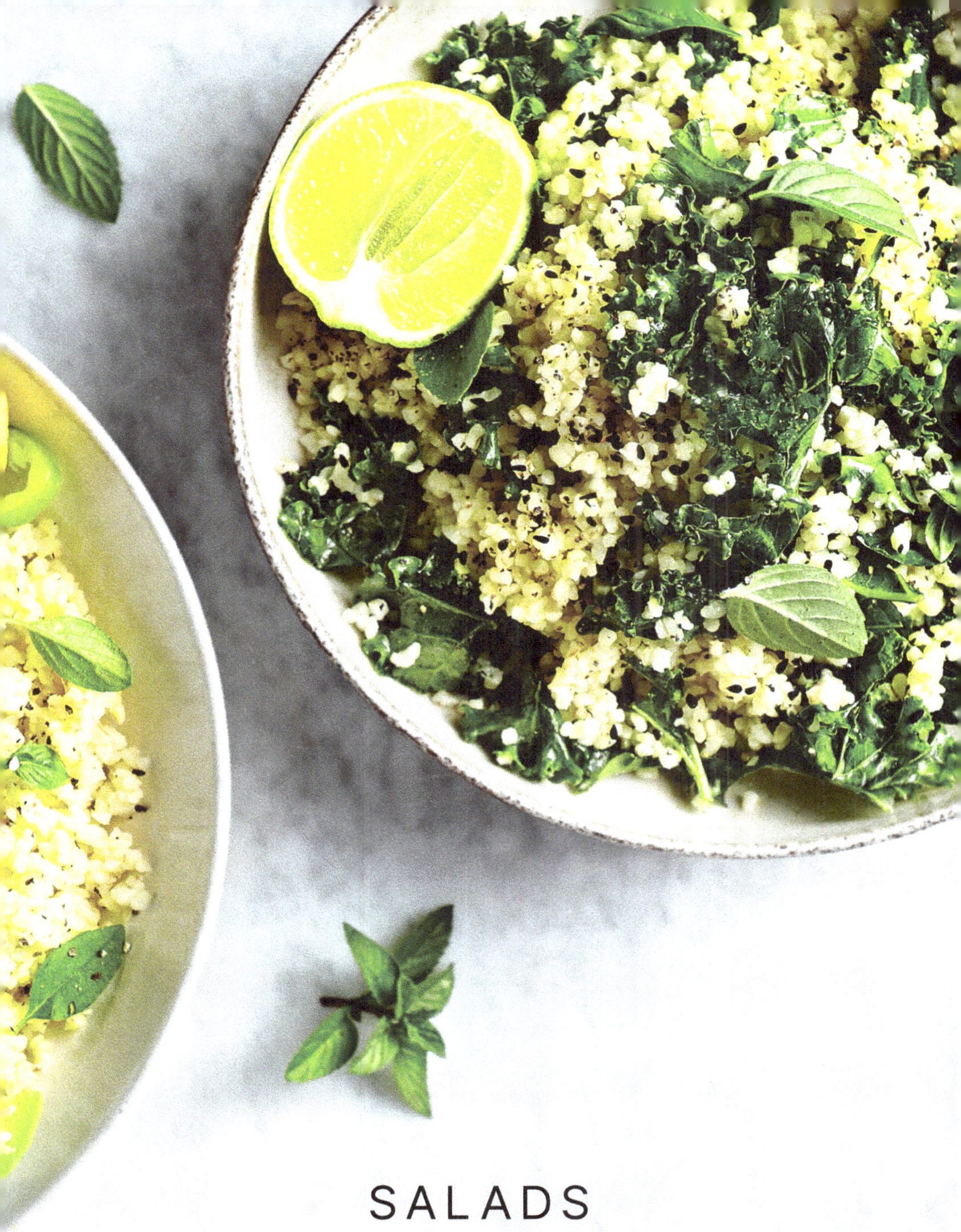

SALADS

Colorful Greek Salad

Serves: 2 **|** *Prep Time: 10 minutes* **|** *Cook Time: 25 resting*

As we covered earlier in the book, the journey to a healing diet does not need to be perfect. The goal is to have a balanced diet as low in processed foods as possible. A great strategy to accomplish this goal is to make your plate as colorful as possible. This is a very simple salad, however, bursting with micronutrients.

The pomegranate is a creative addition that is packed with antioxidants, and the lemon has a good dose of vitamin C, to mention a few. You can have it as a main dish or, to make it a full meal, you could even add the Turmeric Roasted Chickpeas on top.

INGREDIENTS

- 1 large cucumber
- 1 large tomato
- 1 pomegranate
- 1 cup fresh parsley, chopped
- ¼ cup (50 grams) feta per person
- 1–2 medium lemon
- Olive oil, to taste
- Salt and pepper

DIRECTIONS

1. Carefully peel the cucumbers, cut them into two lengthwise, remove their seeds, and mince finely.
2. Place them in a strainer over a bowl, sprinkle with table-salt, and leave them to exude their vegetable moisture for twenty-five minutes.
3. While that is working, chop the tomato, pomegranate (cut open then pull out the seeds), and parsley. Set aside.
4. When the cucumbers are drained, press them in a towel once more, and remove them to the same bowl as the other ingredients.
5. Cut the lemons into wedges. Set aside.
6. Season your salad with pepper, oil, lemon, and add chopped parsley to taste.
7. Plate your salad. Place 1 lemon wedge on the side of each dish for an additional pop of color and flavor.

Nutritional Facts (per serving):	
Disclaimer: *Nutritional values are estimates and may vary by ingredients and preparation.*	
Serves	2
Serving Size	1 plated salad (~350–400 g)
Calories	~210 kcal
Protein	6 g
Carbohydrates	16 g
Fiber	4 g
Sugars	10 g (mostly from pomegranate)
Fats	14 g
Saturated Fat	4 g
Unsaturated Fat	10 g
Sodium	~320 mg
Vitamin A	~25% DV
Vitamin C	~40% DV
Calcium	~15% DV
Iron	~8% DV
Magnesium	~10% DV
Potassium	~500 mg
Antioxidants	High (from pomegranate, parsley, and lemon)

Fruit and Goat Cheese Salad with a Tangy Vinaigrette

Servings: 2 | *Prep Time: 15 minutes*

Some of the best recipes are ones that use flavor combinations you wouldn't have originally thought of. This salad is one of them. It is also a great option because it offers strong micronutrient content, is easy to prepare, and it is delicious—all ideal requirements for a dish you should keep on repeat during your healing journey and beyond. This recipe is also provided for this book courtesy of Registered Dietitian Nutritionist Ilana Muhlstein, author of *Love the Food That Loves You Back*. You can find out more about her work by booking a private session with her, purchasing her cookbook, and following her on social media at @ilanamuhlsteinrd.

INGREDIENTS

Salad

- 4–6 cups spinach
- ¼ cup goat cheese
- ¼ cup fresh mint, chopped
- ¼ cup fresh basil, chopped
- 1 peach, pear, or apple, thinly sliced
- 2 Persian cucumbers, chopped
- ¼ red onion, chopped
- 2 Tbsp dried unsweetened cranberries, roughly chopped
- 2 Tbsp crushed walnuts (optional)

Dressing

- 2 Tbsp balsamic vinegar
- 1 Tbsp rice wine vinegar
- 2 Tbsp olive oil
- 1 Tbsp honey
- 1 Tbsp Dijon mustard
- ½ tsp salt

DIRECTIONS

1. Chop ingredients and add to a large bowl.
2. In a small bowl, whisk ingredients for dressing, then top salad with dressing. Enjoy!

Nutritional Facts (per serving):	
Disclaimer: *Nutritional values are estimates and may vary by ingredients and preparation.*	
Serves	2
Serving Size	~1 large salad (~350–400 g)
Calories	~310 kcal
Protein	7 g
Carbohydrates	22 g
Fiber	4 g
Sugars	14 g (from fruit, honey, and cranberries)
Fats	22 g
Saturated Fat	5 g
Unsaturated Fat	17 g
Sodium	~380 mg
Vitamin A	~90% DV
Vitamin C	~35% DV
Calcium	~15% DV
Iron	~12% DV
Magnesium	~18% DV
Potassium	~650 mg
Antioxidants	High (from spinach, herbs, fruit, cranberries, and balsamic vinegar)

Healthy Tuna Salad

Serves: 4 | *Prep Time: 10 minutes*

This is a high protein, low fat alternative to your average tuna salad. As tuna salad is usually filled with mayonnaise and saturated fat, we instead swap in Greek yogurt here. With the right seasoning, you can hardly tell any difference. This dish is great to prepare in advance (try doubling it) and you have an easy snack or meal waiting in the fridge. You can spoon a portion on top of a salad, a rice bowl, or dip a few crackers in it. The hardest part of this dish is chopping veggies. Once you have them prepared, all you essentially need to do is combine it all. With the healthy fats and protein from the fish, and micronutrients from the veggies, you have an ideal dish to keep you satisfied and nourished in the second half of your recovery.

INGREDIENTS

- 3 5-oz cans of tuna in water
- 1 cup Greek yogurt
- 2 hard boiled eggs
- Half a red onion, diced
- 3 stalks celery, sliced into small pieces
- ½ cucumber, diced
- Juice of ½ a lemon
- 1 tsp salt
- 1 tsp garlic powder
- 1 tsp paprika
- ½ tsp pepper, more to taste
- 2 Tbsp chives, optional

DIRECTIONS

1. Drain the tuna and chop your veggies and eggs.
2. Assemble all in a large bowl, including spices. Mix well.
3. Spread on toast, crackers, or over a bed of greens. Enjoy!

Nutritional Facts (per serving):	
Disclaimer: *Nutritional values are estimates and may vary by ingredients and preparation.*	
Serves	4
Serving Size	~1 heaping cup (~200–220 g)
Calories	~210 kcal
Protein	28 g
Carbohydrates	5 g
Fiber	1 g
Sugars	3 g (from yogurt, onion, and cucumber)
Fats	8 g
Saturated Fat	2 g
Unsaturated Fat	6 g
Sodium	~480 mg (based on added salt and tuna)
Vitamin A	~6% DV
Vitamin C	~10% DV
Calcium	~8% DV
Iron	~10% DV
Magnesium	~10% DV
Potassium	~500 mg
Antioxidants	Moderate (from lemon juice, paprika, cucumber, and red onion)

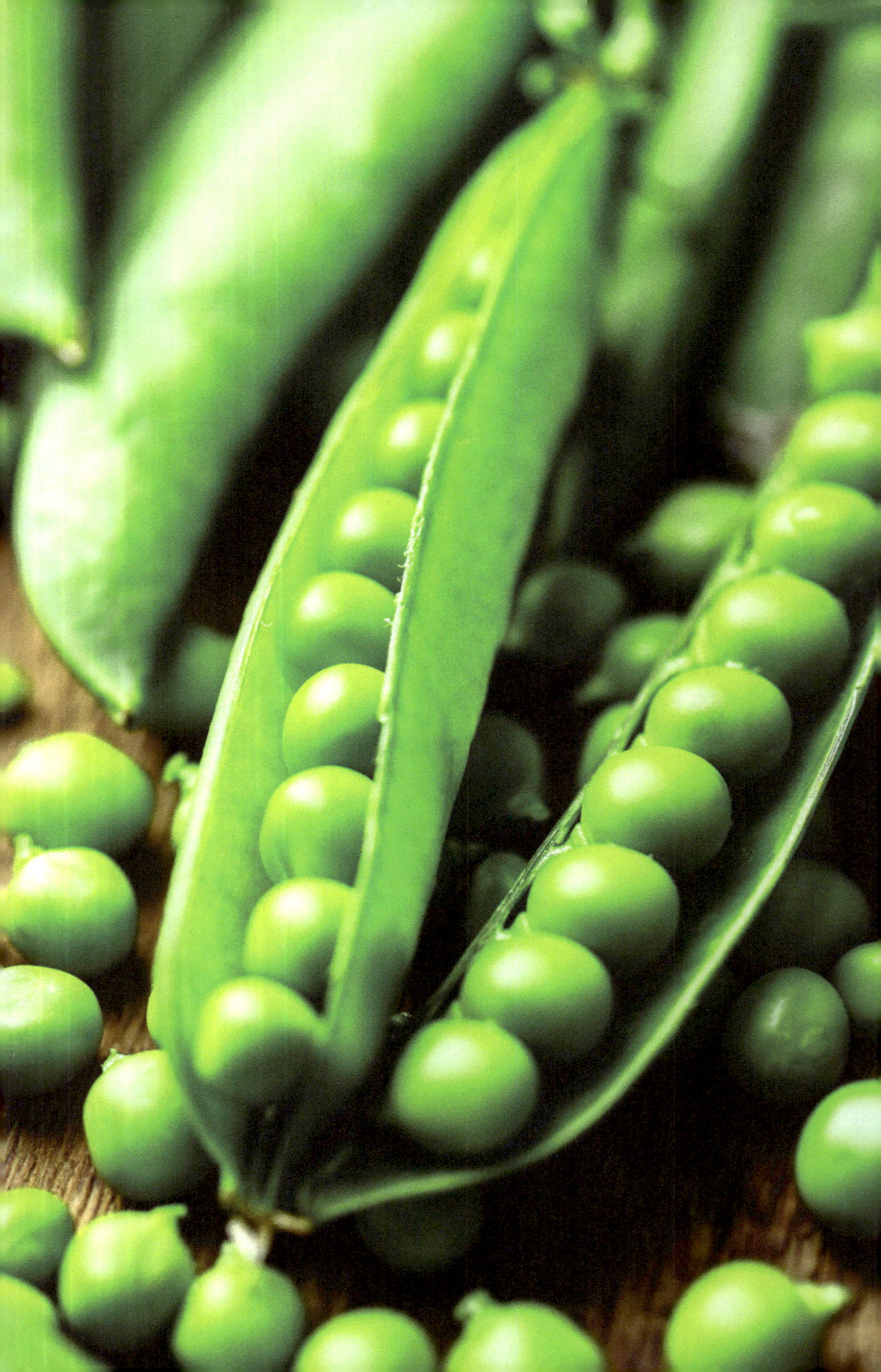

Grilled Citrus Chicken Salad with Tarragon Vinaigrette

Servings: 4 | Prep Time: 10 minutes | Cook Time: 10 minutes

My favorite types of salads not only have a variety of veggies but proteins and fats as well. If you can throw in carbs as well, you have a winner. This salad contains my first two requirements of proteins from the chicken and fats from the dressing. It also has a variety of veggies which makes life more exciting than eating simple lettuce. Also, the dressing contains tarragon which is more unique than your everyday oregano. I bet you don't taste it every day. Don't worry about adding more spaces to your cabinet, however—once you purchase it, you will likely want this salad on repeat and will use it up in no time.

This salad is provided courtesy of Dini Klein, the foodie and creator of Prep + Rally (prepandrally.com). Dini offers meal inspiration if you are aiming to adopt a healthy eating lifestyle. You can find more of her simple, delicious meals by following Dini at @prepandrally on all socials.

INGREDIENTS

Salad

- 12 oz sugar snap peas, each halved on a bias
- 4 ears of corn, cut off the cob
- 3 peaches, cut into 2–3 inch chunks
- 1 small onion, thinly sliced
- 3–4 Tbsp neutral cooking oil
- Salt and pepper to season liberally

Chicken

- Zest and juice of 1 orange (¼ cup juice)
- 1 Tbsp pure maple syrup
- 1 Tbsp neutral cooking oil
- 1½ tsp Dijon mustard
- 1¼ tsp Kosher salt
- ¼ tsp black pepper
- 1½ pounds boneless skinless chicken breasts, cut into 2-inch chunks

Tarragon Vinaigrette

- 1 clove garlic
- 1 Tbsp Dijon mustard
- 1 Tbsp pure maple syrup
- ¼ cup packed tarragon leaves, stems discarded
- ¼ cup rice vinegar
- ¼ cup + 2 Tbsp extra virgin olive oil
- Salt and pepper to season

DIRECTIONS

1. To make the salad, place the snap peas, corn, peaches, and onion in a large bowl. Mix with the oil and season with salt and pepper, tossing to coat. Set aside.
2. In a medium bowl, mix together the orange zest and juice, maple syrup, oil, mustard, salt and pepper. Add the chicken and let marinate for a few minutes while you prepare the vinaigrette and heat the grill.
3. To make the tarragon vinaigrette, place all ingredients into a wide-mouthed storage jar and blend with an immersion blender.
4. Season to taste and set aside for serving.
5. Heat 2 griddles, smooth side, (or grill pans) on medium high heat and let heat for 5 minutes.
6. Add all the salad ingredients to one griddle or pan and the chicken to the other, mixing both around periodically to evenly brown the chicken on all sides, and until the vegetables have softened and charred in spots (around 15 minutes).
7. Once the chicken is mostly cooked, add it to the vegetables and finish cooking all together, mixing everything around until the flavors have combined.
8. Spoon everything into a serving bowl and toss in the tarragon vinaigrette. Serve hot, and enjoy!

Nutritional Facts (per serving):	
Disclaimer: *Nutritional values are estimates and may vary by ingredients and preparation.*	
Serves	4
Serving Size	~1 full bowl (~450–500 g)
Calories	~520 kcal
Protein	34 g
Carbohydrates	32 g
Fiber	5 g
Sugars	19 g (naturally from corn, peaches, and maple syrup)
Fats	30 g
Saturated Fat	4 g
Unsaturated Fat	26 g
Sodium	~550 mg
Vitamin A	~20% DV
Vitamin C	~45% DV
Calcium	~6% DV
Iron	~10% DV
Magnesium	~15% DV
Potassium	~700 mg
Antioxidants	High (from peaches, snap peas, onion, tarragon, and garlic)

Asian Cucumber Salad

Servings: 4 | *Prep Time: 10 minutes*

These next two salads are cucumber focused because in my opinion, cucumber is an underrated veggie. It is a vegetable made primarily of water, therefore excellent to keep you hydrated which we know is beneficial during recovery. Cucumbers are good for digestion and crunchy and fresh veggie to add to your meals. They also contain essential nutrients, including vitamin K, vitamin C, magnesium, potassium, and fiber. Earlier chapters mention the benefits of these vitamins.

INGREDIENTS

- 6 mini cucumbers or 2.5 large
- 1½ Tbsp salt
- 1 Tbsp chili flakes (optional)
- 2 Tbsp rice wine vinegar
- 1 Tbsp honey or sugar
- 2 cloves grated garlic
- 1 tsp sesame oil
- 1 tsp sesame seeds

DIRECTIONS

1. Cut off the ends on each cucumber and slice in half lengthwise. Then into 2 inch segments and smash them until slightly bruised. This will allow more of the marinade to soak in.
2. Add salt and allow the cucumbers to rest for 30 minutes to draw out moisture.
3. Rinse off all the salt thoroughly 1-2 times then dry with a paper towel.
4. Mix the remaining ingredients in a small bowl and combine with cucumbers. For best results, let it marinate for an hour in the fridge.

Nutritional Facts (per serving):	
Disclaimer: *Nutritional values are estimates and may vary by ingredients and preparation.*	
Serves	4
Serving Size	~½ cup (~100–120 g)
Calories	~45 kcal
Protein	1 g
Carbohydrates	5 g
Fiber	1 g
Sugars	2 g (from cucumbers and honey/sugar)
Fats	2.5 g
Saturated Fat	0.3 g
Unsaturated Fat	2.2 g
Sodium	~220 mg (after rinsing salt; varies by rinse effectiveness)
Vitamin A	~6% DV
Vitamin C	~10% DV
Calcium	~2% DV
Iron	~4% DV
Magnesium	~5% DV
Potassium	~200 mg
Antioxidants	High (from garlic, chili flakes, sesame oil, and cucumbers)

Mason Jar Persian Cucumber Salad

Servings: 1–2 | *Prep Time: 10 minutes*

If you can describe a salad as crunchy, salty, and creamy, you have my attention. In my opinion, this salad offers a unique option for someone who wants a light and refreshing salad but is bored of lettuce. The fresh herbs and feta provide a unique flavor combination that is hard to resist, and the latter offers some healthy fat to keep you satisfied. Tossed together with nuts and zesty flavors, it makes eating healthy and clean easier.

INGREDIENTS

- 5–6 Persian cucumbers
- 1 avocado
- 1 scallion
- Fresh dill
- Fresh mint
- Walnuts, toasted
- 1.5 oz feta cheese
- 2 Tbsp sumac
- 1 lemon, zest and juice
- Salt and pepper to taste.

DIRECTIONS

1. Thinly slice or dice five or six Persian cucumbers. Add them to a mason jar or salad bowl.
2. Cube an avocado and add to the jar/bowl.
3. Thinly slice the scallion (both the white and green part), dill, and fresh mint (about ⅓ cup per herb chopped).
4. Add walnuts (or pistachios), feta cheese, and sumac for a nice tangy touch.
5. Dress it up with the zest of a full lemon, lemon juice, olive oil, a couple pinches of salt and pepper.
6. Shake the mason jar or Tupperware, or toss in a bowl.

Nutritional Facts (per serving):	
Disclaimer: *Nutritional values are estimates and may vary by ingredients and preparation.*	
Serves	2
Serving Size	~1 generous salad (~300–350 g)
Calories	~330 kcal
Protein	6 g
Carbohydrates	14 g
Fiber	6 g
Sugars	4 g (naturally from cucumber and scallion)
Fats	28 g
Saturated Fat	6 g
Unsaturated Fat	22 g
Sodium	~350 mg (from feta and seasoning)
Vitamin A	~20% DV
Vitamin C	~30% DV
Calcium	~10% DV
Iron	~10% DV
Magnesium	~20% DV
Potassium	~650 mg
Antioxidants	High (from fresh herbs, lemon zest, sumac, and walnuts)

High Protein Chicken & Bean Salad

Servings: 6 | *Prep Time: 20 minutes*

Beans are often underestimated and not given the attention they deserve as a health food. They contain so many great benefits and cover some of the main nutritional bases: proteins, fats, and carbs. All in one food, you might ask? Correct. That is why this salad is packed with fiber and proteins. As I mentioned, the best salads contain both macro and micronutrients via lean proteins, healthy fats, and veggies. It makes recovery even simpler by having everything on one plate, doesn't it?

INGREDIENTS

Salad

- 1 can white beans
- 1 can cannellini beans
- 1 whole rotisserie chicken, shredded
- 1 medium red onion
- 1 cucumber
- 2 bell peppers (I used orange and yellow)
- ¾ cup kalamata olives
- 9 oz pickled beets
- 7 oz sheep's milk feta
- 8 oz cherry tomatoes

Dressing

- ⅓ cup olive oil
- ⅔ cup sherry vinegar
- ¼ diced parsley
- 1 Tbsp Dijon mustard
- 1 Tbsp honey
- 1 Tbsp Italian seasoning
- Salt and pepper to taste

DIRECTIONS

1. Drain the beans and rinse them. Place in a large bowl.
2. Combine the dressing ingredients and set aside.
3. Cut all the other ingredients into similar sized pieces and add them to the bowl.
4. Combine with the dressing and enjoy!

Nutritional Facts (per serving):	
Disclaimer: *Nutritional values are estimates and may vary by ingredients and preparation.*	
Serves	6
Serving Size	~1½–2 cups (~400–450 g)
Calories	~520 kcal
Protein	32 g
Carbohydrates	28 g
Fiber	7 g
Sugars	7 g (from beets, honey, onion, and peppers)
Fats	30 g
Saturated Fat	8 g
Unsaturated Fat	22 g
Sodium	~720 mg (from olives, feta, and seasoning)
Vitamin A	~25% DV
Vitamin C	~60% DV
Calcium	~20% DV
Iron	~25% DV
Magnesium	~25% DV
Potassium	~850 mg
Antioxidants	Very high (from beets, olives, tomatoes, parsley, and peppers)

Wild Rice Kale Salad

Servings: 6 | Prep Time: 5 minutes | Cook Time: 25 minutes

Packed with nutrient-dense ingredients, this Wild Rice Kale Salad combines the earthy flavors of wild rice with the hearty texture of kale. Rich in fiber, antioxidants, and essential vitamins, this salad promotes digestive health and supports immune function while providing a satisfying crunch. Perfect on its own for snack or lunch, or add grilled chicken or fish for dinner. Would also be great for stuffed bell peppers!

INGREDIENTS

Salad

- 1 cup dry wild rice
- 2 cups water or bone broth
- 1 cup chopped kale
- ½ cup chopped dates or other dried fruit
- ½ cup cashews or nut of choice
- 1 can lentils
- ¼ a red onion, diced
- 3 green onion, chopped
- ¼ cup hemp seeds
- 3 celery stalks, chopped

Dressing

- Juice of 1 lemon
- 2 Tbsp olive oil
- 1 Tbsp red wine vinegar
- 1 Tbsp Dijon
- 1 tsp honey
- Salt and pepper to taste

DIRECTIONS

1. Cook your rice by boiling it in broth for about 20–25 minutes. Let cool while you chop the rest of the ingredients.
2. Make the dressing in a bowl or small mason jar. Toss rice, veggies and dressing and enjoy.

Nutritional Facts (per serving):	
Disclaimer: *Nutritional values are estimates and may vary by ingredients and preparation.*	
Serves	**6**
Serving Size	**~1½ cups (~300–350 g)**
Calories	**~360 kcal**
Protein	**13 g**
Carbohydrates	**37 g**
Fiber	**7 g**
Sugars	**7 g (mostly from dates or dried fruit)**
Fats	**18 g**
Saturated Fat	**2.5 g**
Unsaturated Fat	**15.5 g**
Sodium	**~220 mg (depends on salt added and broth used)**
Vitamin A	**~60% DV**
Vitamin C	**~30% DV**
Calcium	**~10% DV**
Iron	**~20% DV**
Magnesium	**~25% DV**
Potassium	**~650 mg**
Antioxidants	**High (from kale, hemp seeds, dried fruit, red onion, and lemon juice)**

Cabbage Crunch Salad

Servings: 2–4 | Prep Time: 10 minutes

This Cabbage Crunch Salad is a refreshing medley of vibrant cabbage, crunchy vegetables, and tangy dressing. Cabbage is known for its high vitamin C content and anti-inflammatory properties, making this salad a fantastic choice for boosting immunity and overall gut health. If you're like me, you need a crunch in your salad along with different flavors to make it exciting. This provides those satisfying elements to turn a boring salad into one you want to have again and again.

INGREDIENTS

Salad

- 2–3 cups shredded cabbage (or one bag)
- 1 cup shredded carrots (or one small bag)
- 5–6 celery stalks, chopped
- 1 red bell pepper, chopped
- Cilantro or parsley, chopped
- ¼ cup hemp seeds
- ¼ cup pumpkin seeds
- Protein of choice

Dressing

- 5 Tbsp olive oil
- 4 Tbsp apple cider vinegar
- 2 Tbsp honey
- 2 Tbsp minced ginger
- 1 tsp ground turmeric
- Salt + pepper
- Juice of 1 large lemon or 2 small

DIRECTIONS

1. Chop all veggies and herbs. Toss together.
2. Top with avocado and the protein of your choice.

Nutritional Facts (per serving):	
Disclaimer: *Nutritional values are estimates and may vary by ingredients and preparation.*	
Serves	4
Serving Size	~1½–2 cups (~300–350 g)
Calories	~270 kcal
Protein	6 g
Carbohydrates	16 g
Fiber	5 g
Sugars	8 g (from carrots, red bell pepper, and honey)
Fats	21 g
Saturated Fat	2.5 g
Unsaturated Fat	18.5 g
Sodium	~180 mg (depends on added salt)
Vitamin A	~100% DV
Vitamin C	~80% DV
Calcium	~10% DV
Iron	~15% DV
Magnesium	~20% DV
Potassium	~600 mg
Antioxidants	High (from turmeric, ginger, cabbage, bell pepper, lemon juice, and seeds)

Colorful Orzo Salad

Servings: 3–4 | *Prep Time: 10 minutes*

Adding color to your plate will provide a variety of essential micronutrients for healing. This salad is a delicious and fresh option when you want to try something different while nourishing your body. It also proves not all salads are boring! By adding orzo, we get some sustaining carbohydrates to compliment the variety of veggies. It is also nice to note that this is a salad without lettuce, so it will not wilt, which makes it perfect for meal prep. If you want to add extra protein, try adding some grilled chicken.

INGREDIENTS

Salad

- 3 cups cooked orzo
- 1 cup halved cherry tomatoes
- 1 cup diced cucumber
- ½ cup chopped sun dried tomatoes
- ½ cup vegan feta
- 1 cup kalamata olives, chopped or whole
- Garnish with fresh dill

Dressing

- ⅓ cup olive oil
- 3 Tbsp red wine vinegar
- 1 Tbsp whole grain mustard
- 1 Tbsp lemon juice
- 1 tsp each of salt, pepper, oregano, and garlic powder

DIRECTIONS

1. Chop your veggies and whisk together your dressing.
2. Combine in a large bowl or Tupperware and mix well together.
3. If you are meal prepping, separate in portions and refrigerate for up to four days.

Nutritional Facts (per serving):	
Disclaimer: *Nutritional values are estimates and may vary by ingredients and preparation.*	
Serves	4
Serving Size	~1½ cups (~350–400 g)
Calories	~440 kcal
Protein	9 g
Carbohydrates	38 g
Fiber	4 g
Sugars	5 g (mostly from tomatoes and cucumber)
Fats	28 g
Saturated Fat	5 g
Unsaturated Fat	23 g
Sodium	~580 mg (from olives, vegan feta, and seasonings)
Vitamin A	~15% DV
Vitamin C	~25% DV
Calcium	~10% DV
Iron	~12% DV
Magnesium	~10% DV
Potassium	~450 mg
Antioxidants	High (from sun-dried tomatoes, olives, garlic, lemon, and dill)

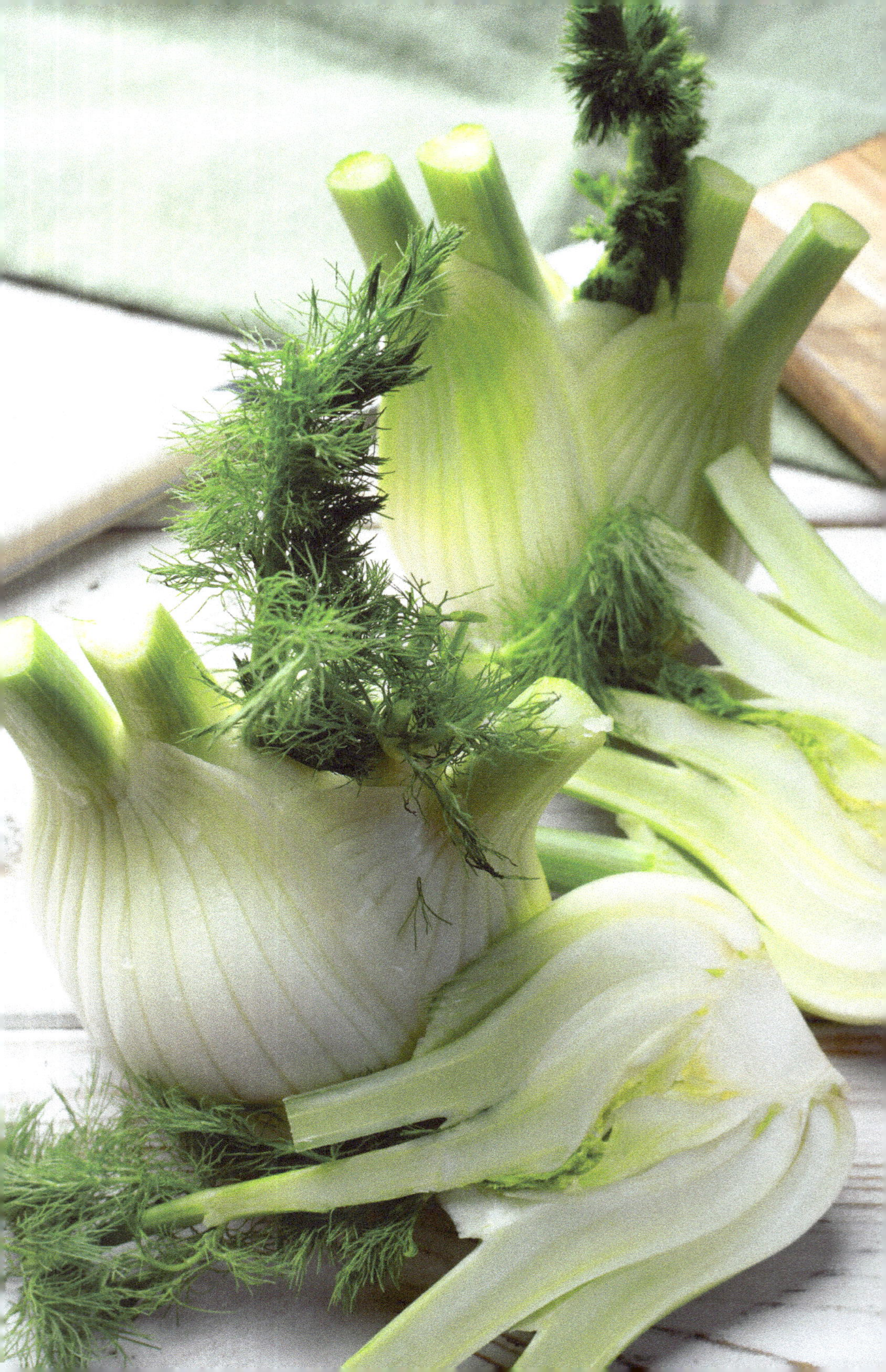

Steak Fennel Salad

Servings: 2 | Cook Time: 15 minutes

As we have discussed throughout the book, proteins and the amino acids that they provide are one of the best building blocks of a healing nutritious diet. You should aim to have about 1 gram per pound of body weight per day, more or less, for optimal results. When you start tracking your protein, you will realize how intentionally you have to be eating to achieve this. Most people do not eat their daily protein goal without proper planning. Also, you will realize how much more satiated you feel by eating lean, whole proteins. This dish is an excellent option when you want something fresh but satisfying.

This salad is a simple but healthy dish by holistic chef Elizabeth Leigh Mandelbaum. There are easy-to-source vibrant flavors in this dish that elevate the experience of a simple salad into a luxurious one. You can purchase her cookbook *Plated* on Amazon which is packed with unique and nutritious recipes. Also, you can discover more of her healthy creations at @elizabethleigh.m on Instagram.

INGREDIENTS

Salad

- 2 oyster steaks (organic, grass fed)
- 16 oz arugula
- 2 fennel plants
- Olive oil
- Salt and pepper

Dressing

- ⅓ cup olive oil
- 2 Tbsp vinegar
- ½ lemon, squeezed
- 1 or 2 cloves garlic, crushed

DIRECTIONS

Steak

1. Remove the steaks from the fridge about 8 minutes before cooking. Using a knife, slash 3 diagonal lines on each side of the filets. Sprinkle salt and pepper on both sides.
2. Heat a skillet or grill pan with 2 tbsp olive oil.
3. Place the steaks down, let them cook for 5–8 minutes on each side. I like to use a tong to press the steaks down on the edges as well to make sure I get an even cook on the meat.

Salad

1. Cut, wash then slice the fennel into super thin slices.
2. Split the arugula in half, placing half on one plate and half on the second plate. Add the fennel to each salad.
3. Assemble the dressing by combining all the dressing ingredients in a bowl and mixing well.
4. Dress the salad then place each steak over the bed greens. Serve and enjoy!

Nutritional Facts (per serving):	
Disclaimer: *Nutritional values are estimates and may vary by ingredients and preparation.*	
Serves	2
Serving Size	1 steak + salad (~400–450 g)
Calories	~520 kcal
Protein	40 g
Carbohydrates	8 g
Fiber	3 g
Sugars	3 g (from fennel and lemon)
Fats	38 g
Saturated Fat	9 g
Unsaturated Fat	29 g
Sodium	~280 mg (depends on added salt)
Vitamin A	~35% DV
Vitamin C	~30% DV
Calcium	~10% DV
Iron	~25% DV
Magnesium	~15% DV
Potassium	~750 mg
Antioxidants	High (from arugula, fennel, garlic, lemon, and olive oil)

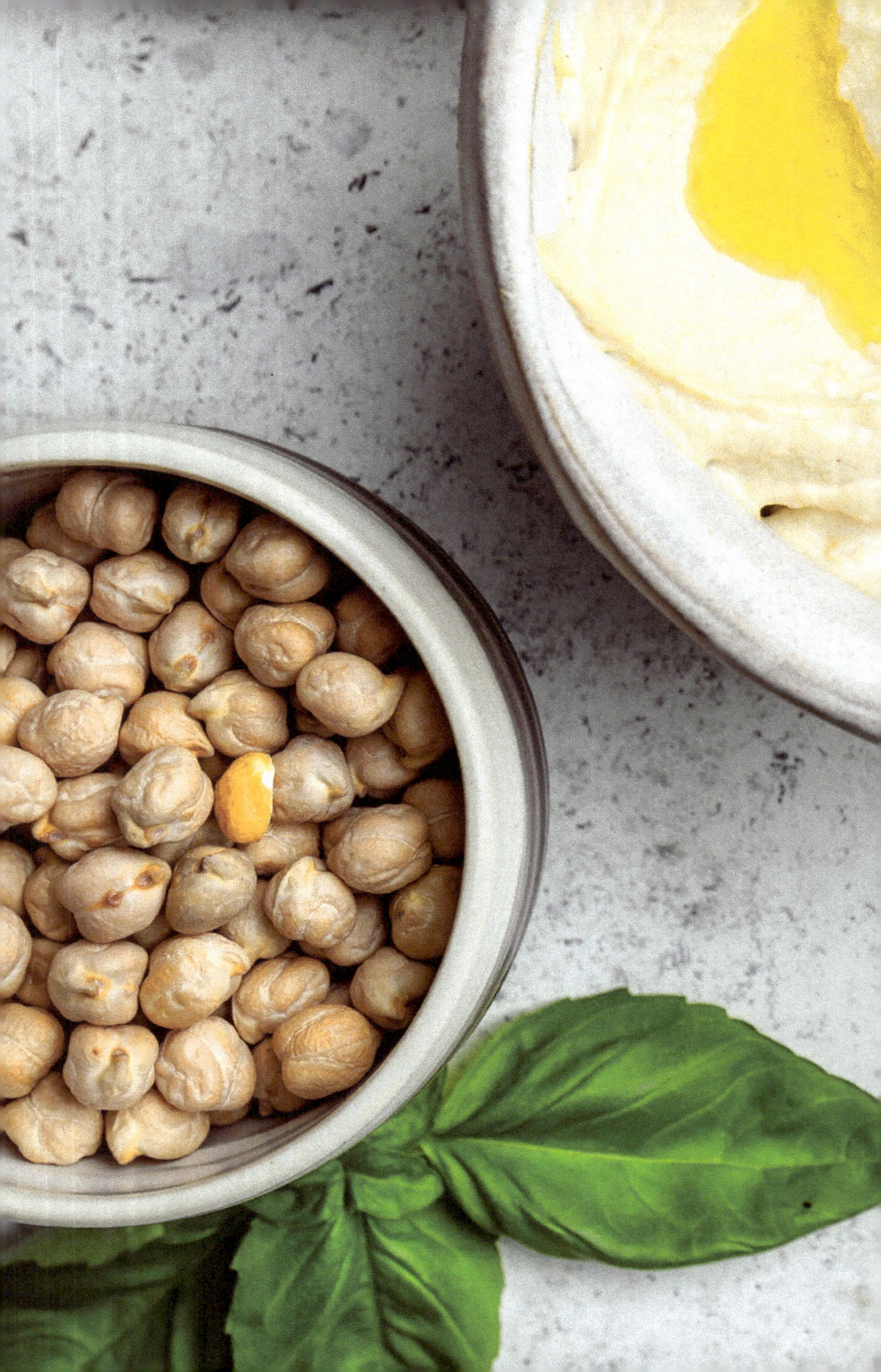

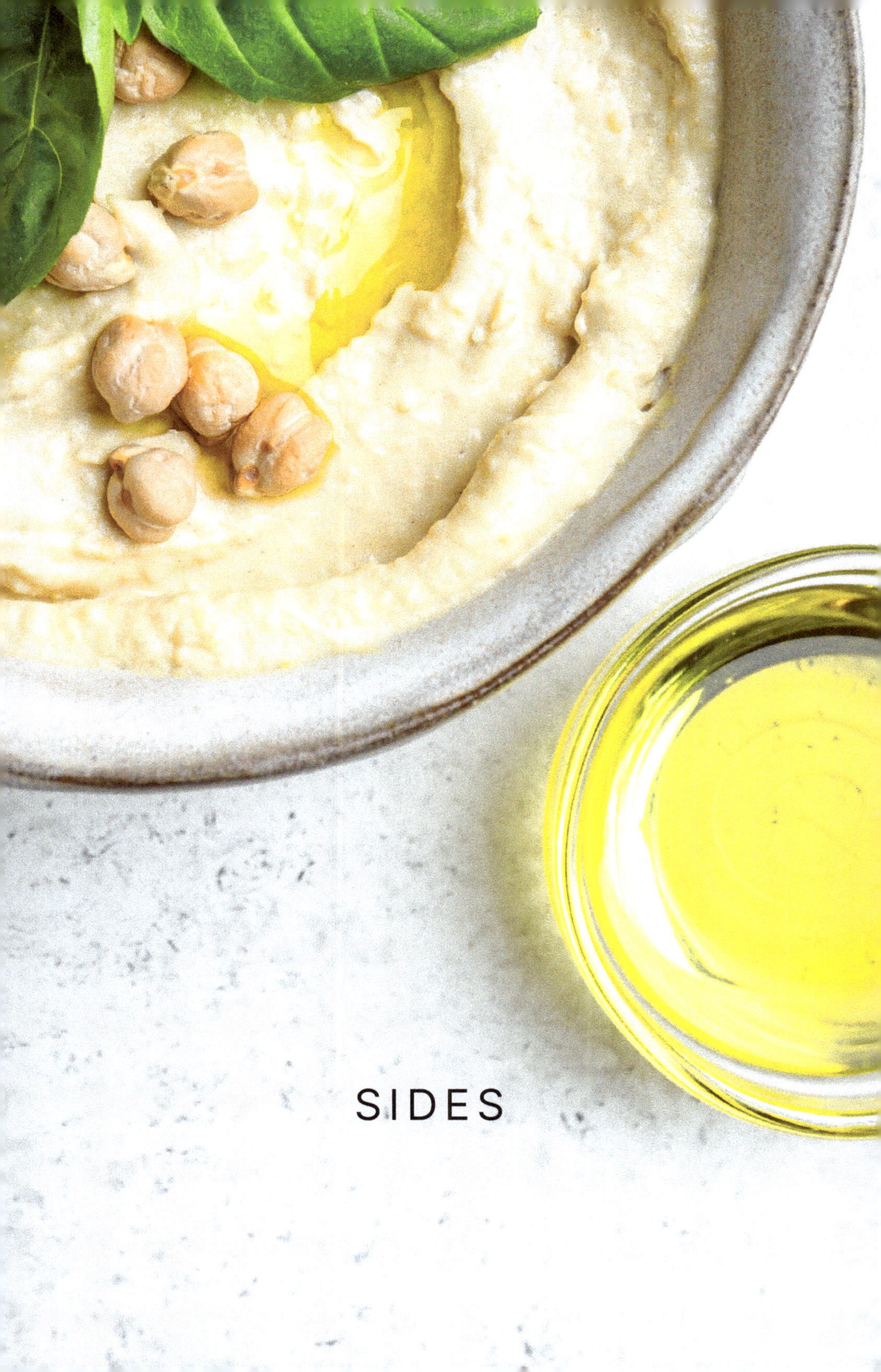

SIDES

Traditional Hummus

Prep Time: 10 minutes

Creamy and flavorful, this hummus is a classic Middle Eastern dip made from chickpeas, tahini, and olive oil. Chickpeas are an excellent source of plant-based protein and fiber, supporting heart health and aiding in digestion while offering a deliciously versatile snack option. While there are many store-bought options, making your own allows you to control what goes inside, as well as create the most cost-effective portions.

This recipe was created by Andrea Amatte, a viral recipe creator with millions of followers across the globe. Andrea creates a variety of international recipes that are healthy and delicious. You can find more of her work at @andrearecetas on Instagram.

INGREDIENTS

- 10 oz of canned chickpeas
- 1 clove garlic
- 1 Tbsp tahini
- Salt to taste
- Pepper to taste
- Cumin to taste (optional)
- Lemon juice to taste
- Olive oil
- Cold water, 2 Tbsp

DIRECTIONS

1. Boil the chickpeas until they are very soft and almost puree. Save the water.
2. Pour the lemon juice along with the tahini into the food processor and process until everything is integrated.
3. Then, add the chickpeas with a little bit of cooking water, the garlic, and the other ingredients.
4. Process very well until you have a super smooth cream. Add very cold water to obtain a much creamier consistency.

Nutritional Facts (per serving):	
Disclaimer: *Nutritional values are estimates and may vary by ingredients and preparation.*	
Serves	2
Serving Size	~½ cup (approx. 130–150 g)
Calories	~250 kcal
Protein	9 g
Carbohydrates	22 g
Fiber	6 g
Sugars	3 g
Fats	14 g
Saturated Fat	2 g
Unsaturated Fat	12 g
Sodium	~220 mg (varies by added salt)
Vitamin C	~10% DV
Calcium	~6% DV
Iron	~15% DV
Magnesium	~18% DV
Potassium	~300 mg

Express Focaccia

Servings: 10 | *Cook Time: 20–25 minutes*

This Express Focaccia is a quick and easy bread recipe that is perfect for pairing with soups or salads. While still a treat, this focaccia can be enhanced with herbs and olive oil, offering heart-healthy fats and satisfying flavors without the long preparation time. This recipe was also created by Andrea Amatte, the talented viral recipe creator who I mentioned on the previous page. You can follow at @andrearecetas on Instagram.

INGREDIENTS

Ferment

- 1¼ cups water
- 2 tsp dry yeast
- 1 tsp sugar

Dough

- 560g all-purpose whole flour
- 1 tsp salt
- 1–2 tsp olive oil for drizzling

DIRECTIONS

Ferment

1. Mix the water with the yeast and sugar. Let it rest for 10 minutes.

Dough

2. In a bowl add the flour, salt, prepared ferment mixture from step 1 and olive oil. Integrate with a spatula and then arrange it a little more with an oiled hand. Let rise covered for 30 or 40 minutes.
3. Then, inside the bowl, make some folds to the dough (as seen in the video) and let it rise again until it doubles in size. Massage briefly to release the air and place on a deep oven-safe plate.

4. Add the dough and press the entire surface with your fingers.
5. You can add cherry tomatoes, rosemary, onion, olives, among others. Finish with a good splash of olive oil and salt.
6. Let it rest again and then bake at 400 degrees F until golden brown. It's a delight!

Nutritional Facts (per serving):	
Disclaimer: *Nutritional values are estimates and may vary by ingredients and preparation.*	
Serves	**10**
Serving Size	**1 slice (~85–90 g)**
Calories	**~210 kcal**
Protein	**6 g**
Carbohydrates	**36 g**
Fiber	**3 g**
Sugars	**1 g (from flour and ferment)**
Fats	**5 g**
Saturated Fat	**0.7 g**
Unsaturated Fat	**4.3 g**
Sodium	**~230 mg**
Vitamin A	**~0% DV**
Vitamin C	**~0% DV (unless toppings added)**
Calcium	**~1% DV**
Iron	**~10% DV**
Magnesium	**~8% DV**
Potassium	**~110 mg**
Antioxidants	**Moderate (enhanced if using herbs, tomatoes, or olives as toppings)**

Versatile Egg White Tortilla

Servings: 4 tortillas | *Prep Time: 5 minutes* | *Cook Time: 8–10 minutes*

The Versatile Egg White Tortilla is a staple that can effortlessly transition between breakfast, lunch, and dinner. These tortillas provide a quick source of energy while being adaptable for numerous nutritious fillings, making them a healthy option all week long. To praise its additional benefits, it is both gluten free and sugar free. Just like any wrap, you can make the fillings sweet or salty. This recipe was also created by Andrea Amatte, the talented viral recipe creator behind the food recipe platform @andrearecetas on Instagram.

INGREDIENTS

- 4 egg whites
- Salt to taste
- Splash of vanilla extract
- Sesame seeds, for topping

DIRECTIONS

1. Preheat the oven to 350 degrees F (175 degrees C). Line a baking sheet with parchment paper.
2. Beat egg whites with salt and vanilla until stiff peaks form.
3. Spoon into rounds on parchment; sprinkle sesame seeds.
4. Bake until set and lightly golden, 8–10 minutes.
5. Cool slightly, then fill as desired.

Nutritional Facts (per serving):	
Disclaimer: *Nutritional values are estimates and may vary by ingredients and preparation.*	
Serves	**4**
Serving Size	**1 filled wrap (~100–120 g depending on fillings)**
Calories	**~45 kcal (without fillings)**
Protein	**9 g**
Carbohydrates	**~0.5 g**
Fiber	**0 g**
Sugars	**0 g**
Fats	**1 g**
Saturated Fat	**0.3 g**
Unsaturated Fat	**0.7 g**
Sodium	**~110 mg (from egg whites + salt)**
Vitamin A	**~0% DV**
Vitamin C	**~0% DV**
Calcium	**~1% DV**
Iron	**~2% DV**
Magnesium	**~1% DV**
Potassium	**~100 mg**
Antioxidants	**Low (unless enhanced by fillings like bell pepper and greens)**

Low Carb Coconut Bread

Servings: 10 | Prep time: 10 min | Cook time: 45 min

Ideal for those following a low-carb or ketogenic diet, Keto Coconut Bread is low in carbs yet high in flavor. Even if you are not, there are some great healing recipes that are keto. Made primarily from coconut flour, this bread is rich in healthy fats and fiber, helping to keep you fuller longer while providing a guilt-free bread alternative. If you want to have this always ready to eat, make two batches and slice the bread before you freeze it.

INGREDIENTS

- 6 medium eggs (or 5 extra large)
- 1 Tbsp coconut oil
- ¾ cup coconut Flour
- 1 tsp baking powder
- Pinch of salt
- ½ tsp or less of xanthan gum (optional, to have a more sticky bread)

DIRECTIONS

1. Mix all dry ingredients in a big bowl.
2. Add the whole eggs and the coconut oil.
3. Mix well with a spoon until it gets thick. You can add extra coconut flour if you feel it is too liquid.
4. Preheat your oven to 350 degrees F (175 degrees C).
5. Pour the dough evenly into a Bread/Loaf form (coated with butter or parchment paper) and cook for 35 to 45 minutes.
6. After cooking, remove it from the oven and let it sit while it cools down.
7. Some variations can be done, like using butter instead of coconut oil or adding pumpkin puree to the mix and having a cake-like texture.

Nutritional Facts (per serving):	
Disclaimer: *Nutritional values are estimates and may vary by ingredients and preparation.*	
Serves	10
Serving Size	1 slice (~40–45 g)
Calories	~125 kcal
Protein	5 g
Carbohydrates	4 g
Fiber	3 g
Sugars	1 g (naturally from coconut and eggs)
Fats	9 g
Saturated Fat	7 g
Unsaturated Fat	2 g
Sodium	~130 mg
Vitamin A	~4% DV
Vitamin C	0% DV
Calcium	~3% DV
Iron	~6% DV
Magnesium	~6% DV
Potassium	~90 mg
Antioxidants	Moderate (from coconut flour and eggs)

Protein Flatbread

Serves: 1–2 | Cook time: 30 minutes

Protein is one of the key micronutrients in your healing journey. When you are feeling more recovered and eager to try new recipes, this is a standard you can customize over and over again. It is a healthier version of pizza, a golden comfort food, but made with higher protein ingredients. The cottage cheese is the secret ingredient, but combined with the eggs and cheese, you have yourself a protein filled meal before you even get to the toppings. You can add chickpeas, sliced ham, or whatever additional protein you desire. The same goes for veggie toppings.

INGREDIENTS

- 1 cup cottage cheese
- 2 eggs
- ½ cup marinara sauce
- ½ cup mozzarella
- ¼ cup Parmesan cheese
- Toppings of your choice

DIRECTIONS

1. Preheat your oven to 325 degrees F and prepare a baking sheet. Add a Tbsp of olive oil and wipe it across the sheet. It is essential to oil the entire sheet to prevent any part of the flatbread from sticking.
2. Combine the cottage cheese and eggs together in a blender until smooth.
3. Pour the mixture onto the sheet. Using a spatula, shape it either in rectangle or circle, to your preference.
4. Bake for 15 minutes. Remove it from the oven and add marinara sauce and mozzarella cheese on top.
5. Insert it back into the oven for another 10 minutes.
6. Remove one last time to add toppings and Parmesan. Bake for another 5 minutes.
7. Remove from the oven and let it cool slightly (helps it firm up). Enjoy!

Nutritional Facts (per serving):	
Disclaimer: *Nutritional values are estimates and may vary by ingredients and preparation.*	
Serves	2
Serving Size	½ flatbread (~200–225 g with sauce and cheese)
Calories	~290 kcal
Protein	26 g
Carbohydrates	6 g
Fiber	1 g
Sugars	3 g (from marinara and dairy)
Fats	17 g
Saturated Fat	8 g
Unsaturated Fat	9 g
Sodium	~550 mg
Vitamin A	~12% DV
Vitamin C	~4% DV (depends on toppings)
Calcium	~25% DV
Iron	~6% DV
Magnesium	~8% DV
Potassium	~250 mg
Antioxidants	Moderate (from marinara and any veggie toppings)

Crispy Carrots with Yogurt Dressing

Servings: 4 | Prep Time: 5 minutes | Cook Time: 25 minutes

Crispy Carrots with Yogurt Dressing is a deliciously wholesome snack or side dish that highlights the natural sweetness of carrots. Rich in beta-carotene and vitamins, this recipe promotes healthy vision and skin, while the yogurt dressing adds a creamy, probiotic boost. When cooked right, carrots can taste better than they get credit for. It is an underrated root vegetable that has many vitamins and benefits to the body, and it is also very versatile. You can put it in juices or make it savory like this recipe does as a side dish.

INGREDIENTS

Base

- 1 lb carrots, sliced into 3-inch long flat pieces
- ½ cup extra-virgin olive oil
- ½ cup grated Parmigiano Reggiano (split into 2 ¼-cups)
- 1 tsp onion powder
- 1 tsp cumin
- 1 tsp paprika
- 1 tsp salt
- 1 tsp chili flakes
- Sea salt to taste

Yogurt Dressing

- 4 Tbsp plain Greek yogurt
- 1 garlic clove, pressed
- ½ lemon, juice
- ¼ cup milk

DIRECTIONS

1. Preheat the oven to 425 degrees F.
2. In a bowl, add onion powder, cumin, paprika, salt, chili flakes, and olive oil. Mix well and coat the carrot pieces. Add ¼ cup Parmigiano Reggiano and toss.
3. Place the carrot sticks evenly on a baking tray and add a layer of Parmigiano Reggiano on top.
4. Bake in the oven for 20–25 minutes or until tender. Remove, plate, and sprinkle on some salt.

5. In a separate bowl, add the yogurt dressing ingredients and whisk until smooth.
6. Drizzle yogurt dressing on the carrots and finish with a sprinkle of paprika and cumin. Enjoy!

Nutritional Facts (per serving):	
Disclaimer: *Nutritional values are estimates and may vary by ingredients and preparation.*	
Serves	**4**
Serving Size	**~1 cup (~200–225 g carrots with dressing)**
Calories	**~250 kcal**
Protein	**5 g**
Carbohydrates	**13 g**
Fiber	**4 g**
Sugars	**6 g (naturally from carrots and milk)**
Fats	**20 g**
Saturated Fat	**5 g**
Unsaturated Fat	**15 g**
Sodium	**~430 mg**
Vitamin A	**~320% DV**
Vitamin C	**~15% DV**
Calcium	**~15% DV**
Iron	**~6% DV**
Magnesium	**~10% DV**
Potassium	**~550 mg**
Antioxidants	**Very high (from carrots, paprika, cumin, and garlic)**

Plant Based Cashew Cheese

Servings: About 1–2 cups | *Prep Time: 5 minutes*

As mentioned earlier in this book, you should try to avoid dairy in your healing diet, as it can be inflammatory, with the exception of Greek yogurt. Processed cheeses, however, could contain preservatives and high amounts of unhealthy fat and salt. This cashew cheese is a great alternative to satisfy any cheesy cravings and can be eaten as a dip, or added on top of bowls, tacos, or burritos. The nuts provide healthy fats and minerals, along with some protein as well.

INGREDIENTS

- 1 cup cashews
- 1 cup hot water
- 1 Tbsp harissa paste and/or chili crunch
- 2 Tbsp nutritional yeast
- Salt and pepper to taste

DIRECTIONS

1. Add ingredients in a blender and blend until smooth, adding a bit more water if needed.
2. Pair it with your favorite crudités or drizzle on top of a bowl or wrap.

Nutritional Facts (per serving):	
Disclaimer: *Nutritional values are estimates and may vary by ingredients and preparation.*	
Serves	**6**
Serving Size	**~2–3 tablespoons (~45–50 g)**
Calories	**~140 kcal**
Protein	**4 g**
Carbohydrates	**8 g**
Fiber	**1 g**
Sugars	**1 g (naturally from cashews)**
Fats	**11 g**
Saturated Fat	**2 g**
Unsaturated Fat	**9 g**
Sodium	**~120 mg (varies with harissa/chili crunch)**
Vitamin A	**~2% DV**
Vitamin C	**~1% DV**
Calcium	**~1% DV**
Iron	**~6% DV**
Magnesium	**~15% DV**
Potassium	**~150 mg**
Antioxidants	**Moderate to high (from chili paste, garlic, and nutritional yeast)**

Upside Down Parmesan Sweet Potatoes

Servings: 2–4 | Prep Time: 5 minutes | Cook Time: 30–40 minutes

This unique Upside Down Parmesan Sweet Potatoes dish beautifully combines the sweetness of the potatoes with the savory flavor of Parmesan. Sweet potatoes are rich in vitamin A and antioxidants, making them a nutritious side dish that supports eye health and reduces inflammation. I am always looking for ways to make classic dishes more interesting. These sweet potatoes offer a fun and interesting approach to something you might love but be tired of doing the same old way.

INGREDIENTS

- 4 small sweet potatoes, cut in half lengthwise
- 2 Tbsp olive oil
- ½ tsp garlic powder
- ½ tsp Italian seasoning or other spice blend
- ½ cup finely shredded Parmesan cheese
- Chopped scallion for topping (optional)
- Olive or chili oil for topping (optional)

DIRECTIONS

1. Preheat your oven to 400 degrees F and prepare a baking sheet.
2. In a bowl, season your cut sweet potatoes with olive oil and spices until well coated.
3. Shred Parmesan cheese onto your baking sheet and spread so that it's evenly coated.
4. Place sweet potatoes cut-side down on top of the Parmesan.
5. Bake for 30–40 minutes until sweet potatoes are tender and the bottom layer of cheese is crispy.
6. Let cool for a few minutes. Top with herbs and oil and enjoy.

Nutritional Facts (per serving):	
Disclaimer: *Nutritional values are estimates and may vary by ingredients and preparation.*	
Serves	4
Serving Size	~½ sweet potato (~200–225 g cooked with cheese)
Calories	~210 kcal
Protein	4 g
Carbohydrates	25 g
Fiber	4 g
Sugars	6 g (naturally from sweet potatoes)
Fats	11 g
Saturated Fat	3 g
Unsaturated Fat	8 g
Sodium	~250 mg (from cheese and seasoning)
Vitamin A	~300% DV
Vitamin C	~15% DV
Calcium	~10% DV
Iron	~6% DV
Magnesium	~12% DV
Potassium	~500 mg
Antioxidants	High (from sweet potatoes, herbs, and optional chili oil)

Baba Ganoush

Servings: 4 **|** *Cook Time: 30 minutes*

Smokey and savory, baba ganoush is a traditional Middle Eastern eggplant dip that is both flavorful and healthy. Eggplant is low in calories and high in fiber, making this dip not only a delicious accompaniment but also a great choice for weight management and digestive support. This recipe also comes with a secret ingredient: yogurt, which gives it a unique creaminess! This recipe was also created by Andrea Amatte, the talented viral recipe creator behind the food recipe platform @andrearecetas on Instagram.

INGREDIENTS

- 2 eggplants
- 1 clove garlic
- Salt to taste
- Pepper to taste
- Olive oil to taste
- 1 Tbsp lemon juice
- 1 Tbsp tahini
- 1 Tbsp yogurt

DIRECTIONS

1. Roast whole eggplants in a 400 degrees F (200 degrees C) oven until skin chars and flesh softens, about 30 minutes.
2. Let cool; scoop out pulp.
3. In a food processor, blend pulp with garlic, tahini, yogurt, lemon juice, and seasonings until smooth.
4. Transfer to a bowl; swirl in olive oil, garnish, and serve.

Nutritional Facts (per serving):	
Disclaimer: *Nutritional values are estimates and may vary by ingredients and preparation.*	
Serves	4
Serving Size	~¼ cup (~100–120 g)
Calories	~110 kcal
Protein	2 g
Carbohydrates	7 g
Fiber	3 g
Sugars	3 g (naturally from eggplant and yogurt)
Fats	9 g
Saturated Fat	1.5 g
Unsaturated Fat	7.5 g
Sodium	~100 mg (varies with added salt)
Vitamin A	~2% DV
Vitamin C	~8% DV
Calcium	~4% DV
Iron	~5% DV
Magnesium	~6% DV
Potassium	~300 mg
Antioxidants	High (from eggplant skin, garlic, lemon, and parsley)

Turmeric Roasted Chickpeas

Servings: 4 | *Prep Time: 5 minutes* | *Cook Time: 45 minutes*

Turmeric Roasted Chickpeas are a crunchy, flavorful snack rich in plant-based protein and anti-inflammatory properties. The addition of turmeric offers a host of health benefits, including improved digestion and reduced inflammation, making these chickpeas a healthy snack option. What more could one ask for? The fact that it is plant-based is a nice bonus if you have any vegetarians in your household. This dish can be eaten alone, over a salad, or with grain and veggies in a bowl. It is a great dish to meal prep for the week as well.

As I mentioned earlier in the book, turmeric should not be taken prior to surgery. However, afterwards it will help in your recovery due to its strong anti-inflammatory properties. Not to mention, it adds a nice earthy taste to any dish.

INGREDIENTS

- 1 can (15 oz) chickpeas, drained and rinsed
- 1 Tbsp olive oil
- 1 tsp turmeric powder
- ½ tsp cumin
- Salt to taste

DIRECTIONS

1. Preheat the oven to 400 degrees F.
2. Dry the chickpeas with a paper towel and place them in a bowl.
3. Add olive oil, turmeric, cumin, and salt. Toss to coat.
4. Prepare parchment paper over a flat rectangular pan for the oven and evenly spread out the chickpeas over the paper.
5. Cook in the oven for about 45 minutes, checking on them and shaking the pan about halfway.

Nutritional Facts (per serving):	
Disclaimer: *Nutritional values are estimates and may vary by ingredients and preparation.*	
Serves	4
Serving Size	~⅓ cup (~50–60 g)
Calories	~160 kcal
Protein	6 g
Carbohydrates	20 g
Fiber	5 g
Sugars	1 g (naturally from chickpeas)
Fats	6 g
Saturated Fat	1 g
Unsaturated Fat	5 g
Sodium	~180 mg (depends on added salt)
Vitamin A	~1% DV
Vitamin C	~2% DV
Calcium	~4% DV
Iron	~10% DV
Magnesium	~12% DV
Potassium	~250 mg
Antioxidants	High (from turmeric, cumin, and olive oil)

Muhammara

Servings: 6 | *Prep Time: 5 minutes*

This vibrant Muhammara combines roasted red peppers, walnuts, and spices to create a delicious dip that's rich in flavor and nutrients. Packed with healthy fats and antioxidants from walnuts, this Middle Eastern dip supports heart health and is a perfect accompaniment to fresh vegetables or whole grain crackers. This recipe was also provided for this book courtesy of Andrea Amatte, the talented viral recipe creator behind the food recipe platform @andrearecetas on Instagram.

INGREDIENTS

- 1½ roasted and/or fresh peppers
- 1 clove garlic
- 1 cup walnuts, toasted (more if you want more texture in the sauce)
- 2 Tbsp breadcrumbs
- 1 tsp ground cumin
- ½ tsp paprika
- Salt and pepper to taste
- 1 Tbsp lemon juice
- 6 Tbsp (100 ml) extra virgin olive oil

DIRECTIONS

1. In a food processor, blend peppers, garlic, breadcrumbs, walnuts, lemon juice, olive oil and spices until a coarse paste forms.
2. With the motor running, drizzle in olive oil until smooth but still textured. Refrigerate before serving.

Nutritional Facts (per serving):	
Disclaimer: *Nutritional values are estimates and may vary by ingredients and preparation.*	
Serves	6
Serving Size	~2–3 tablespoons (~45–50 g)
Calories	~190 kcal
Protein	3 g
Carbohydrates	5 g
Fiber	1.5 g
Sugars	1.5 g (naturally from peppers)
Fats	18 g
Saturated Fat	1.5 g
Unsaturated Fat	16.5 g
Sodium	~180 mg
Vitamin A	~10% DV
Vitamin C	~30% DV
Calcium	~2% DV
Iron	~6% DV
Magnesium	~10% DV
Potassium	~200 mg
Antioxidants	High (from red peppers, garlic, walnuts, olive oil, and lemon juice)

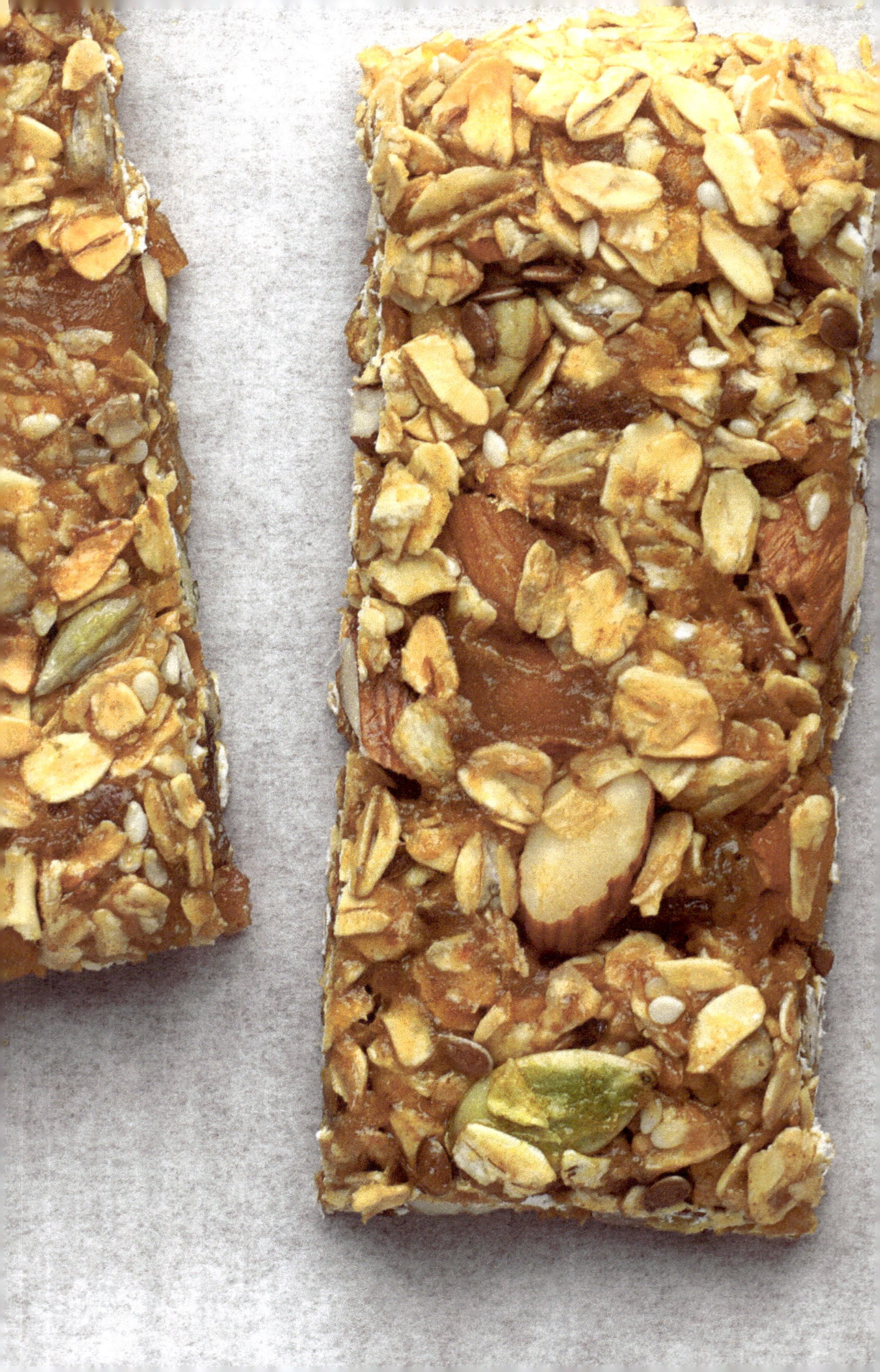

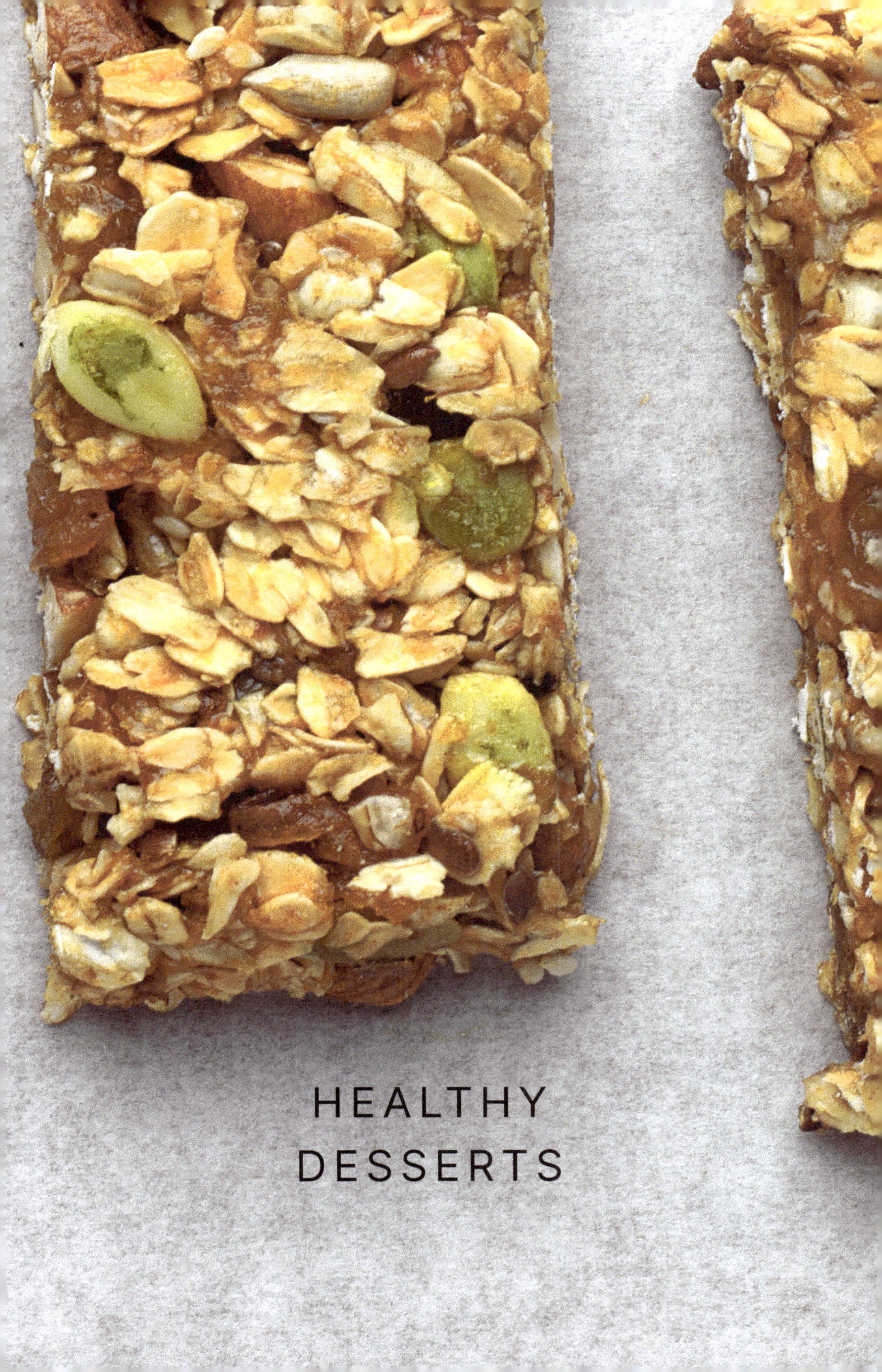

HEALTHY DESSERTS

Strawberry Protein Parfait

Servings: 4 **|** *Prep Time: 10 minutes*

If you have not noticed by now, Greek yogurt is a secret ingredient in many recipes that have been made healthier. This gelato also uses it which adds a boost of high protein and gut-healthy probiotics.

INGREDIENTS

- 1 cup Greek yogurt
- 6–8 medium strawberries, whole
- 6–8 medium strawberries, diced
- 2–3 Tbsp monk fruit sweetener (or honey)
- Splash of vanilla extract
- Handful of chocolate chips and pistachios for topping (optional)

DIRECTIONS

1. Add cottage cheese and Greek yogurt to a food processor or blender.
2. Toss in the whole strawberries, sweetener, and vanilla.
3. Blend until smooth. Taste and adjust if needed.
4. Dice your other 6–8 strawberries.
5. In 4 separate cups, layer a spoonful of diced strawberries, then a couple spoonfuls of the creamy mix. Repeat 1–2 more times.
6. Top with melted sugar-free chocolate and a sprinkle of pistachios (optional).
7. Seal the jars, let them chill, and enjoy it cold!

Nutritional Facts (per serving):	
Disclaimer: *Nutritional values are estimates and may vary by ingredients and preparation.*	
Serves	4
Serving Size	~1 parfait (~150–170 g)
Calories	~180 kcal
Protein	12 g
Carbohydrates	11 g
Fiber	2 g
Sugars	6 g (naturally from strawberries and yogurt; sweetener not included)
Fats	10 g
Saturated Fat	3 g
Unsaturated Fat	7 g
Sodium	~50 mg
Vitamin A	~2% DV
Vitamin C	~60% DV
Calcium	~15% DV
Iron	~4% DV
Magnesium	~8% DV
Potassium	~250 mg
Antioxidants	High (from strawberries, pistachios, and chocolate)

Healthy Granola Bars

Servings: 12 | *Freeze Time: 30 minutes*

Perfect for a quick snack, these bars give a satisfying sweet crunch. Oats and nuts provide fiber and healthy fats. Also, peanut butter is a great source of protein and healthy fats as well, making this treat a nutritious option that provides sustained energy. While regular granola bars are often filled with unnecessarily long ingredient lists, this one has just a few. Another positive aspect is you can customize the fruit (or chocolate) topping depending on your mood.

INGREDIENTS

Base

- 2 cup old-fashioned rolled oats
- ¾ cup roughly chopped nuts like almonds, walnuts, pecans, peanuts or a mix
- ¼ cup sunflower seeds or pepitas or additional chopped nuts
- ¼ cup unsweetened coconut flakes
- ½ cup honey
- ⅓ cup creamy peanut butter
- 2 tsp pure vanilla extract
- ½ tsp ground cinnamon
- ¼ tsp kosher salt

Optional Topping

- ⅓ cup dried strawberries
- ⅓ cup dark chocolate chips
- ⅓ cup dried cranberries

DIRECTIONS

1. Preheat your oven to 325 degrees F. Line a 8x8 or 9x9 square baking dish with parchment paper. Coat lightly with coconut oil.
2. Spread the oats, nuts, sunflower seeds, and coconut flakes on a rimmed, ungreased baking sheet. Toast in the oven until the coconut looks lightly golden and the nuts are toasted and fragrant, about 10 minutes, stirring once halfway through. Reduce the oven temperature to 300 degrees F.
3. In another pan, heat the honey and peanut butter together until the mixture is smooth. Remove from the heat. Stir in the vanilla, cinnamon, and salt.
4. As soon as the oat mixture is finished toasting, carefully transfer it to the pan with the peanut butter. Stir to combine.

5. Let it cool for 5 minutes, then add the chocolate chips (or dried fruit of choice).
6. Scoop the batter into the parchment-lined 8x8 or 9x9 pan. Press the bars until flat.
7. Bake for 15 to 20 minutes (15 for chewy, 20 for crunchy).
8. Let them cool completely in the pan. Remove once cool and cut the bars evenly with a long knife. Enjoy!

Nutritional Facts (per serving):	
Disclaimer: *Nutritional values are estimates and may vary by ingredients and preparation.*	
Serves	**12**
Serving Size	**1 bar (~45–50 g)**
Calories	**~240 kcal**
Protein	**5 g**
Carbohydrates	**25 g**
Fiber	**3 g**
Sugars	**14 g (mostly from honey and dried fruit)**
Fats	**13 g**
Saturated Fat	**3 g**
Unsaturated Fat	**10 g**
Sodium	**~80 mg**
Vitamin A	**~0% DV**
Vitamin C	**~1% DV**
Calcium	**~4% DV**
Iron	**~6% DV**
Magnesium	**~10% DV**
Potassium	**~200 mg**
Antioxidants	**Moderate to high (from nuts, oats, dark chocolate, and berries)**

5-Ingredient Apple Cake

Servings: 2–3 | Prep Time: 5 minutes | Cook Time: 20–30

The easier the recipe, the more I tend to gravitate towards it. It might be a reaction to being very busy and living in an overstimulated world, however, I appreciate recipes with minimal ingredients more and more as time passes. As the title says, this recipe contains only five ingredients, and all of them are very basic ingredients you probably already have in your kitchen. This recipe is great because it contains protein from the cottage cheese and egg, along with micronutrients from the apple. This creates a simple but yummy apple cake that is perfect for breakfast, or even dessert if you are in the mood.

INGREDIENTS

- 1 apple, peeled and cored
- 8 oz cottage cheese
- 1 large egg
- ⅓ cup sweetener (ex: Stevia, allulose, honey, or maple syrup)
- ½ tsp vanilla extract
- Dark chocolate, melted (optional, for topping)

DIRECTIONS

1. Preheat your oven to 350 degrees F.
2. Blend all ingredients in a blender or food processor. With your oil of choice, grease a muffin tin or 2–3 individual ramekins. Pour into 2-3 oven tin slots or ramekins.
3. Bake for 20–30 minutes, testing with a fork or toothpick to ensure it comes out clean.
4. Remove from the oven, add your favorite toppings, and enjoy!

Nutritional Facts (per serving):	
Disclaimer: *Nutritional values are estimates and may vary by ingredients and preparation.*	
Serves	2
Serving Size	~1 small ramekin or slice (~175–200 g) with Stevia & no chocolate
Calories	~180 kcal
Protein	16 g
Carbohydrates	10 g
Fiber	1 g
Sugars	7 g (naturally from apple and cottage cheese)
Fats	8 g
Saturated Fat	3.5 g
Unsaturated Fat	4.5 g
Sodium	~320 mg
Vitamin A	~6% DV
Vitamin C	~4% DV
Calcium	~12% DV
Iron	~4% DV
Magnesium	~6% DV
Potassium	~250 mg
Antioxidants	Moderate (can be increased with dark chocolate topping)

Protein Bars with Chocolate Drizzle

Servings: 16 bars | Prep Time: 15 minutes

When you have a sweet tooth like I do, baking these bars is essential for weekly meal prep. They are full of healthy fats, Omega-3s, fiber, and protein, so they make a great choice over store-bought bars which can contain preservatives, high sugar, and fillers. With the natural sweetness of the dates, the chocolate, and protein powder, it truly feels like eating a dessert but without the guilt. Enjoy this delightful dessert that supports your health goals while satisfying your sweet tooth.

INGREDIENTS

- 2 cup rolled oats
- 1 cup almonds
- 1 cup cashew nut
- ½ cup pumpkin seeds
- 3 cup dates
- 2 scoops protein powder (flavor of choice)
- 1 cup almond butter
- ⅓ cup dark chocolate, melted with 1 tsp coconut oil

DIRECTIONS

1. Toast your oats, almonds, nuts, and seeds in a medium pan over medium heat.
2. Remove any pits from your dates and process them in a food processor or blender until a smooth paste.
3. In another pan, combine the almond butter, date paste, and protein powder. Melt together.
4. Combine the melted paste with the nut and seed mixture and make sure it is evenly coated.
5. Pour into a rectangular sheet-lined pan and pat it firmly down.
6. Drizzle with dark chocolate and refrigerate for at least 1 hour.
7. Cut into bars and enjoy!

Nutritional Facts (per serving):	
Disclaimer: *Nutritional values are estimates and may vary by ingredients and preparation.*	
Serves	16
Serving Size	1 bar (~55–60 g)
Calories	~260 kcal
Protein	10 g
Carbohydrates	24 g
Fiber	4 g
Sugars	14 g (naturally from dates and chocolate)
Fats	15 g
Saturated Fat	3 g
Unsaturated Fat	12 g
Sodium	~50 mg
Vitamin A	~0% DV
Vitamin C	~1% DV
Calcium	~6% DV
Iron	~10% DV
Magnesium	~20% DV
Potassium	~300 mg
Antioxidants	High (from dark chocolate, nuts, and dates)

Sweet Potato Brownies

Serves: 9 | *Prep Time: 10 minutes* | *Cook Time: 20 minutes*

These brownies are a deliciously rich treat that incorporates the natural sweetness and fiber of sweet potatoes. Packed with nutrients and lower in refined sugars, these brownies offer a healthier alternative to brownies from a box, while providing energy and essential vitamins. When starting a healthier lifestyle, people mistakenly think this means no desserts, no joy in life. This is, of course, untrue—you simply need to try out alternative desserts that have healthier ingredients and lower amounts of refined sugars and fillers that could cause inflammation. Enjoy this healthier alternative without the guilt!

INGREDIENTS

- 1 medium sweet potato
- ⅓ cup of cacao powder
- ¼ cup almond or coconut flour
- 1 tsp baking soda
- Pinch of sea salt
- 2 medium eggs
- ¼ cup of nut butter of your choice
- ¼ cup of maple syrup or honey
- 3 Tbsp of coconut oil
- ½ tsp of vanilla extract
- ½ cup of chocolate chips, plus extra for topping

DIRECTIONS

1. Cook the sweet potato according to your preferred method. In the microwave, 5–8 minutes on medium-high. In a pot of boiling water, boil for about 15 minutes or until tender. If in an oven, poke holes in your potato and bake for about 30–40 minutes.
2. Take the skin off the potato (careful not to burn yourself) and mash the interior in a bowl.
3. Add the rest of the ingredients and mix well together.
4. Prepare a baking sheet in a 8x8 pan and pour in the mixture. Top off with extra chocolate chips (and another sprinkle of sea salt if you like; optional).
5. Bake at 350 degrees F for 20 minutes. Check if ready by inserting a fork; it is done if it comes out without batter sticking to it.
6. Remove the pan when ready, let it cool for at least 5–10 minutes, and enjoy!

Nutritional Facts (per serving):	
Disclaimer: *Nutritional values are estimates and may vary by ingredients and preparation.*	
Serves	9
Serving Size	1 brownie (~75–80 g)
Calories	~210 kcal
Protein	4 g
Carbohydrates	23 g
Fiber	4 g
Sugars	13 g (mostly from maple syrup, sweet potato, and chocolate chips)
Fats	12 g
Saturated Fat	5 g
Unsaturated Fat	7 g
Sodium	~120 mg
Vitamin A	~80% DV
Vitamin C	~2% DV
Calcium	~6% DV
Iron	~8% DV
Magnesium	~10% DV
Potassium	~250 mg
Antioxidants	High (from cacao, chocolate chips, and sweet potato)

Chocolate Covered Strawberry Froyo

Servings: 6–8 | Prep Time: 10 minutes | Freeze Time: About 1–2 hours

Ice cream is one of those special sweets that most people have a weakness for, myself included. However, store-bought versions tend to have high sugar and fat, along with many filler ingredients. While this option is more of a frozen yogurt, it hits the spot just the same. The minimal ingredients make it a quick and economical option to make as well. The fresh strawberries and dark chocolate also offer more micronutrients than your typical ice cream. And lets not forget about the high protein content of the yogurt, offering some macros in the mix too.

INGREDIENTS

- 1½ cups strawberries, diced
- 1 cup Greek yogurt
- 1 Tbsp maple syrup
- 1 cup dark chocolate chips
- 2 Tbsp coconut oil

DIRECTIONS

1. Dice your strawberries and combine evenly with the yogurt and syrup.
2. On a baking sheet, serve a palm sized portion of yogurt mixture. Freeze for at least 1–2 hours.
3. Once frozen yogurt is ready, melt the chocolate in a saucepan or microwave on low.
4. Dip each frozen yogurt ball into the chocolate and replace on the sheet. Freeze again for about 5–10 minutes and enjoy.

Nutritional Facts (per serving):	
Disclaimer: *Nutritional values are estimates and may vary by ingredients and preparation.*	
Serves	8
Serving Size	1 bite (~60–70 g each)
Calories	~160 kcal
Protein	4 g
Carbohydrates	14 g
Fiber	2 g
Sugars	10 g (from strawberries, yogurt, maple syrup, and chocolate)
Fats	10 g
Saturated Fat	6 g
Unsaturated Fat	4 g
Sodium	~20 mg
Vitamin A	~2% DV
Vitamin C	~25% DV
Calcium	~8% DV
Iron	~6% DV
Magnesium	~8% DV
Potassium	~200 mg
Antioxidants	High (from strawberries and dark chocolate)

Snickers Frowhoa

Servings: 1 | Prep Time: 5 minutes | Freeze Time (Optional): 1–2 hours

This creamy, satisfying froyo takes inspiration from a Snickers bar but uses only whole, nutrient-rich ingredients—no added sugars, gums, or artificial flavorings. With gut-friendly zucchini, natural peanut butter, and a hint of sweetness from banana and dates, this froyo delivers protein, fiber, and indulgent flavor without spiking your blood sugar.

INGREDIENTS

- ¾ cup unsweetened almond milk (or oat/coconut milk)
- 1 cup frozen peeled zucchini
- ½ frozen banana (for natural sweetness & creaminess)
- ½ scoop (approx. 2 Tbsp) chocolate protein powder
- 2 Tbsp natural peanut butter (or 1½ Tbsp peanut butter powder)
- 1 Medjool date (or omit or halve for even lower sugar)
- 1 tsp cacao powder (optional, for rich chocolate flavor)
- Optional topping: ½ Tbsp crushed roasted peanuts

Directions

1. Add all ingredients to a high-speed blender.
2. Blend until smooth and creamy. Taste and adjust sweetness if needed.
3. Serve immediately for a soft-serve texture.
4. For firmer, scoopable texture, freeze for 1–2 hours, then let soften 5 minutes before scooping.

Nutritional Facts (per serving):	
Disclaimer: *Nutritional values are estimates and may vary by ingredients and preparation.*	
Serving Size	~1 smoothie (~350–400 ml)
Calories	~420 kcal
Protein	23 g
Carbohydrates	40 g
Fiber	~6 g
Sugars	~19 g (entirely from banana and 1 Medjool date)
Fats	~23 g
Saturated Fat	~3 g
Unsaturated Fat	~20 g
Sodium	~250 mg
Vitamin A	~8% DV
Vitamin C	~30% DV
Calcium	~15% DV
Iron	~15% DV
Magnesium	~20% DV
Potassium	~650 mg
Antioxidants	High (from cacao, zucchini, and date)

Easy Yummy Pie

Servings: 8 **|** *Prep Time: 5 minutes* **|** *Cook Time: 40 minutes*

This Easy Yummy Pie is a delightful dessert that combines simplicity with deliciousness. With a crust made from wholesome ingredients, this pie comes with a blend of flavors that makes it an enjoyable, nutrient-rich option for family gatherings or special occasions. This recipe is also provided for this book courtesy of Registered Dietitian Nutritionist Ilana Muhlstein, author of *Love the Food That Loves You Back*. You can find out more about her work by booking a private session with her, purchasing her cookbook, and following her on social media at @ilanamuhlsteinrd.

INGREDIENTS

- 1½ cups whole wheat or gluten free flour
- 1 tsp baking powder
- ¾ cup coconut sugar, or equivalent quantity of natural low-calorie sweetener
- 1 egg
- ½ cup melted coconut oil
- ½ tsp vanilla
- 1 16-oz bag of frozen wild blueberries or 1-lb container of fresh blueberries or 4–5 sliced apples (or combine both blueberries and apples)

DIRECTIONS

1. Preheat the oven to 350 degrees F. Add all of the ingredients except the fruit to a bowl and mix well to form the dough.
2. Spray a pie dish with oil. Spread ¾ of the dough on the bottom of the dish. Use your hands to press the dough down and make an even crust. Add blueberries or apples on top of the crust.
3. Using your fingers, crumble the remaining ¼ dough and scatter along the top of the fruit.
4. Bake for 40 minutes and enjoy.

Nutritional Facts (per serving):	
Disclaimer: *Nutritional values are estimates and may vary by ingredients and preparation.*	
Serves	8
Serving Size	1 slice (~120–130 g)
Calories	~280 kcal
Protein	3 g
Carbohydrates	32 g
Fiber	4 g
Sugars	16 g (naturally from fruit and coconut sugar)
Fats	16 g
Saturated Fat	12 g
Unsaturated Fat	4 g
Sodium	~60 mg
Vitamin A	~2% DV
Vitamin C	~10% DV
Calcium	~3% DV
Iron	~6% DV
Magnesium	~8% DV
Potassium	~200 mg
Antioxidants	Very high (especially with wild blueberries)

NOTE

If using sweet red apples, add the juice of half a lemon to bring some tartness to the dish and help prevent browning.

Frozen Peanut Butter Banana Cubes

Servings: 8 | *Prep Time: 5 minutes* | *Freeze Time: 1–2 hours*

This is another minimal-ingredient recipe that takes only a handful of minutes to put together. There are only four main ingredients, three if you take out the syrup. If you use the monk fruit "maple syrup" alternative, you remove the additional sugars from the equation that would normally be present in traditional maple syrup. I think it is essential to always have a healthy sweet treat on hand if you have a sweet tooth, to avoid caving into packaged options which can contain additives. Since these are already frozen, you can store them in the freezer and remove a portion at room temperature for a few minutes when you are in the mood for sweetness.

INGREDIENTS

- 1 cup Greek yogurt
- 1 Tbsp monk fruit maple syrup, Lakanto brand preferred
- 1 banana
- 4 Tbsp peanut butter
- Nuts for topping
- A silicone ice tray or other mold

DIRECTIONS

1. Mix the syrup in the yogurt and set aside.
2. In a silicone mold, evenly add the peanut butter to the bottom.
3. Then layer it with a slice of banana. For the third layer, cover with yogurt.
4. Freeze for at least 2 hours, pop out of the mold, and enjoy.

Nutritional Facts (per serving):	
Disclaimer: *Nutritional values are estimates and may vary by ingredients and preparation.*	
Serves	8
Serving Size	1 bite (~45–50 g)
Calories	~120 kcal
Protein	5 g
Carbohydrates	7 g
Fiber	1 g
Sugars	3 g (naturally from banana and yogurt; monk fruit adds no sugar)
Fats	8 g
Saturated Fat	2 g
Unsaturated Fat	6 g
Sodium	~40 mg
Vitamin A	~1% DV
Vitamin C	~4% DV
Calcium	~6% DV
Iron	~3% DV
Magnesium	~8% DV
Potassium	~200 mg
Antioxidants	Moderate (from banana and optional nuts)

Super Food Power Cookies

Servings: 8–10 | Prep Time: 10 minutes | Cook Time: 22 minutes

Cookies are definitely a favorite of mine, who doesn't love them? Making them at home allows you to control the sugar and ingredients, and this one includes some of the healthiest ones. You will also get a good dose of fiber and healthy fats from this cookie. The amount of healthy ingredients should remove all guilt from indulging in this delightful snack.

INGREDIENTS

- 4 bananas, mashed
- 1 cup ground flaxseed
- 1½ Tbsp chia seeds
- 6 Tbsp nut butter
- Cinnamon to taste
- Dark chocolate chunks to taste

DIRECTIONS

1. Preheat the oven to 350 degrees F and prepare a baking sheet.
2. In a large bowl, mash bananas. Add flaxseed, chia seeds, peanut butter and a few shakes of cinnamon. Mix together well. Fold in dark chocolate chips/chunks (about ⅓ cup recommended).
3. Drop batter by rounded Tbsp onto parchment paper lined cookie sheet and bake in the oven for about 22 minutes.
4. Enjoy now and store the rest in an airtight container in the fridge for the crazy busy upcoming week.

Nutritional Facts (per serving):	
Disclaimer: *Nutritional values are estimates and may vary by ingredients and preparation.*	
Serves	16
Serving Size	1 cookie (~40 g)
Calories	~120 kcal
Protein	3 g
Carbohydrates	13 g
Fiber	3 g
Sugars	6 g (naturally from banana and chocolate)
Fats	7 g
Saturated Fat	2 g
Unsaturated Fat	5 g
Sodium	~10 mg
Vitamin A	~1% DV
Vitamin C	~4% DV
Calcium	~4% DV
Iron	~6% DV
Magnesium	~10% DV
Potassium	~200 mg
Antioxidants	High (from flax, chia, banana, and dark chocolate)

Healthier Hazelnut Spread

Servings: About 1–2 cups of spread | *Prep Time: 5 minutes*

While this is one of those comfort foods that should be enjoyed in small amounts, enjoy it you should! However, store-bought hazelnut spreads tend to have large amounts of sugar and fat. This recipe has less of that, and instead offers healthier fats than typical. This would be perfect to spread on top of the oats or chia seed puddings in this book.

INGREDIENTS

- 1¼ organic macadamia nuts
- ¼ organic maple syrup
- 1 Tbsp organic cold pressed coconut oil
- 2 Tbsp organic unsweetened cocoa powder
- 1 Tbsp organic cocoa butter
- Pinch of sea salt

DIRECTIONS

1. Blend macadamias in a blender, adding a splash of water.
2. Add maple and coconut oil and blend.
3. Next, add cocoa powder, cocoa butter, and salt. Blend.
4. Add a bit more water if needed for creaminess.

Nutritional Facts (per serving):	
Disclaimer: *Nutritional values are estimates and may vary by ingredients and preparation.*	
Serves	6
Serving Size	~2 tablespoons (~35–40 g)
Calories	~210 kcal
Protein	2 g
Carbohydrates	10 g
Fiber	2 g
Sugars	6 g (from maple syrup)
Fats	20 g
Saturated Fat	7 g
Unsaturated Fat	13 g
Sodium	~30 mg
Vitamin A	~0% DV
Vitamin C	~0% DV
Calcium	~2% DV
Iron	~6% DV
Magnesium	~10% DV
Potassium	~120 mg
Antioxidants	High (from cocoa, macadamias, and maple syrup)

Almond Date Balls

Servings: About 12 balls **|** *Prep Time: 5–10 minutes* **|** *Freeze Time: 3 hours*

Always having a healthy sweet snack in your fridge removes the temptation to grab packaged foods that can potentially slow down your healing by causing inflammation. These easy, minimal-ingredient balls are the ideal option to have ready, and to mention more benefits, they are high in fiber and healthy fats. You can eat them on their own, crumble a few on top of yogurt, or meal prep these and store some in the freezer for the future. You can have a ready-to-eat sweet treat by defrosting them at room temperature, transferring them from the freezer to the fridge the day before, or defrosting a couple minutes in the microwave on low power.

This sweet recipe is by holistic chef Elizabeth Leigh Mandelbaum, a foodie content creator with a focus on clean and simple ingredients. Her work is excellent for a whole-food focused diet like we have been talking about throughout the book. I highly recommend you try her recipes in this book, the ones posted on social media, and the recipes in her cookbook Plated.

INGREDIENTS

- 1 cup raw dates, pits removed
- 1 cup raw almonds
- 1 Tbsp natural almond butter
- 1 tsp vanilla extract

DIRECTIONS

1. Place all 4 ingredients into a blender together and blend for 2 minutes, or until fully combined and smooth. The texture you're looking for is very smooth.
2. Then take a spoonful at a time from the mixture to form little balls. Place the ready balls on a baking sheet lined with parchment paper.
3. Freeze for at least 3 hours then store frozen and serve chilled.

Nutritional Facts (per serving):	
Disclaimer: *Nutritional values are estimates and may vary by ingredients and preparation.*	
Serves	12
Serving Size	1 ball (approx. 25 g)
Calories	~120 kcal
Protein	3 g
Carbohydrates	12 g
Fiber	2.5 g
Sugars	9 g (natural from dates)
Fats	7 g
Saturated Fat	0.5 g
Unsaturated Fat	6.5 g
Sodium	~1 mg
Calcium	~4% DV
Iron	~4% DV
Magnesium	~10% DV
Potassium	~150 mg

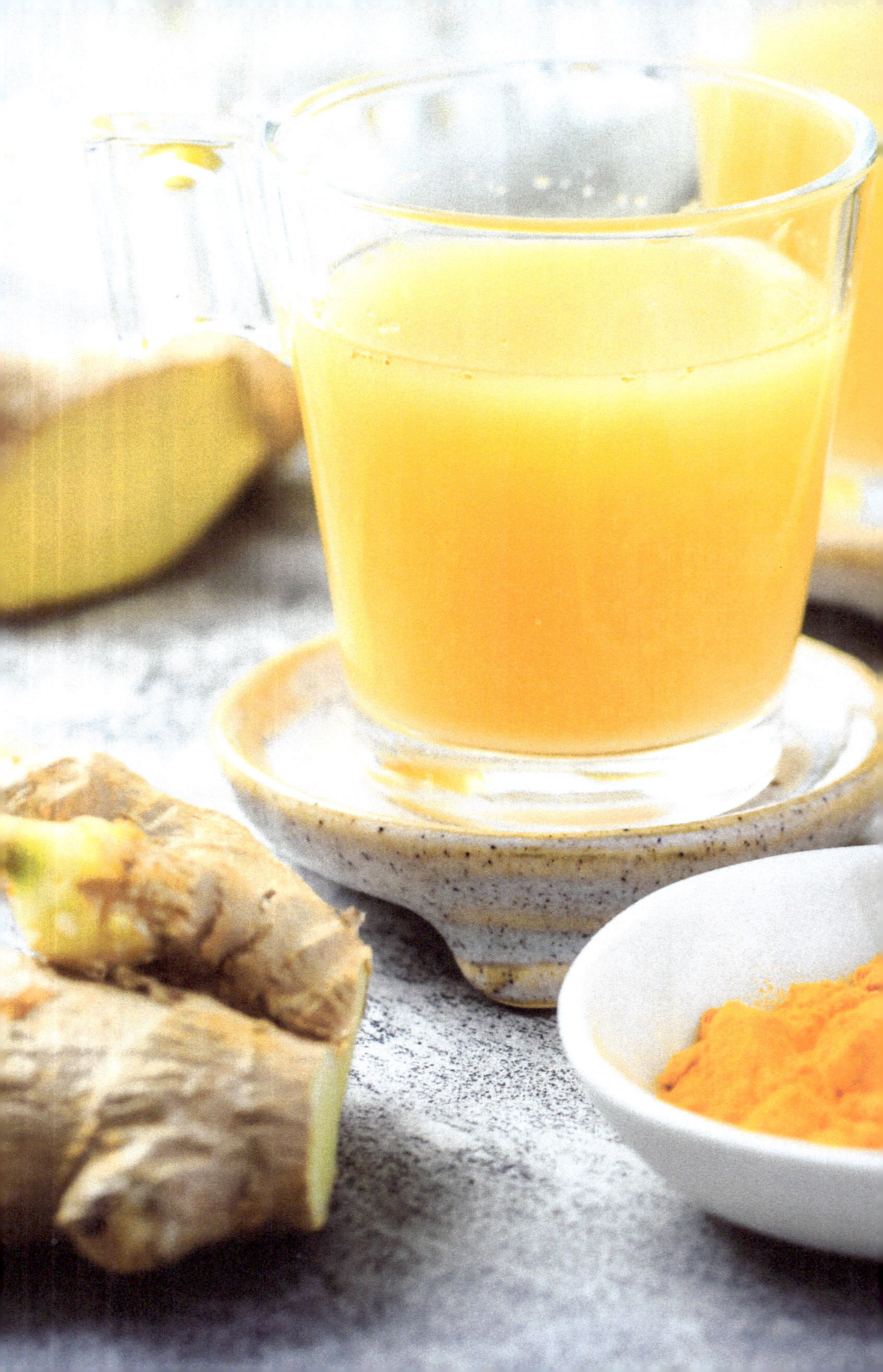

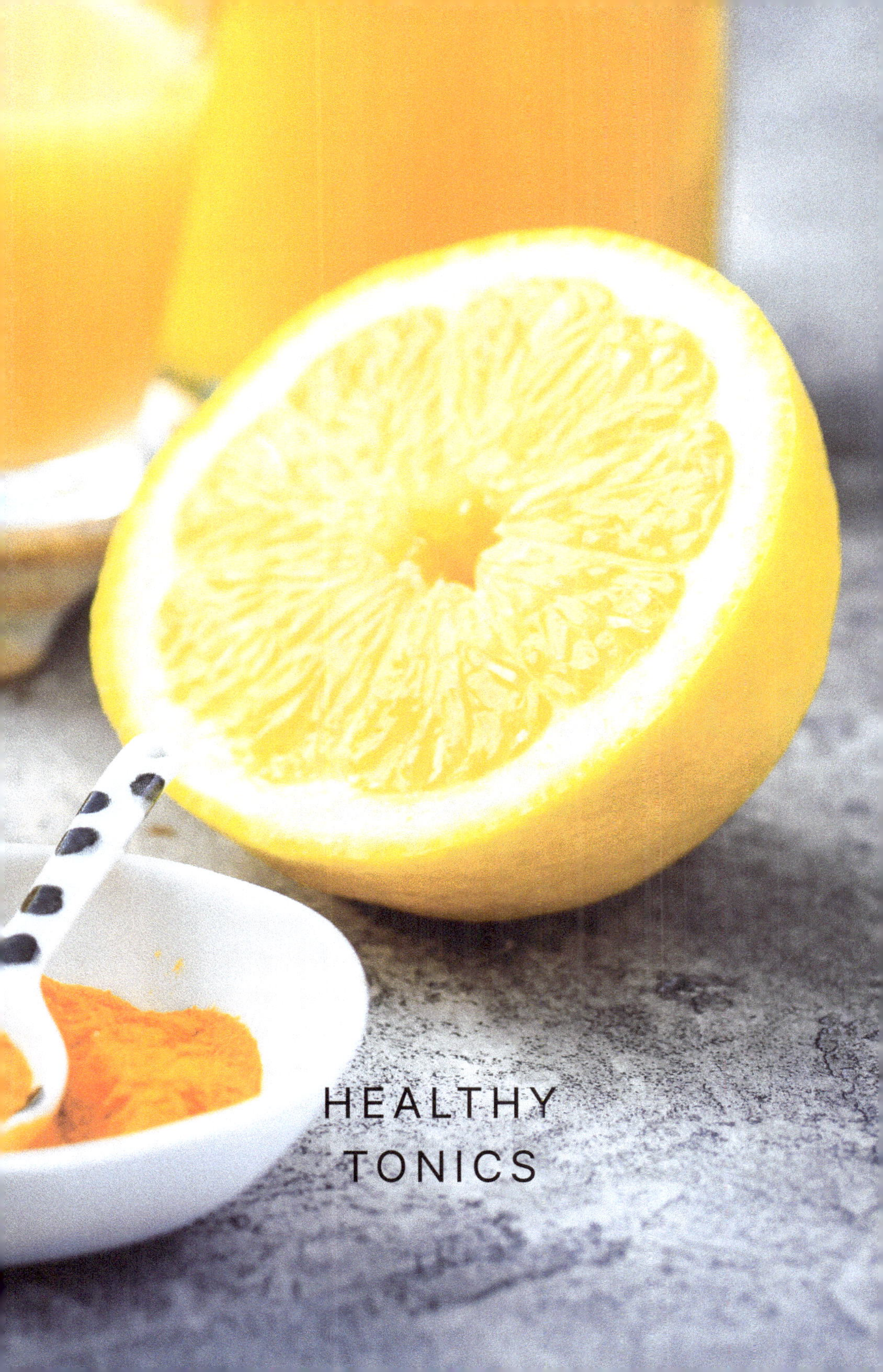

HEALTHY TONICS

Anti-Inflammatory Golden Tonic

Servings: 2 | Prep Time: 5 minutes

Discover the soothing and health-boosting benefits of this refreshing beverage crafted with a harmonious blend of natural ingredients. We combine filtered water and green tea for antioxidants, fresh thyme for its medicinal properties, and grated ginger and turmeric known for their anti-inflammatory effects, this tonic is gently sweetened with Manuka honey and balanced with a splash of raw unfiltered cider vinegar. Served over ice and topped with chilled sparkling water, garnished with lime wedges, it offers a vibrant and revitalizing way to support overall wellness and soothe inflammation.

INGREDIENTS

- 2 cups filtered water
- 2 green tea bags
- 1 sprig of fresh thyme
- 1-inch piece fresh ginger, peeled and grated (~1 tsp)
- 1-inch piece fresh turmeric, peeled and grated (~1 tsp)
- 1 Tbsp raw apple cider vinegar (with the mother)
- 2 tsp manuka or raw honey (adjust to taste)
- 1 cup chilled sparkling water
- Ice cubes
- Chilled sparkling water
- 2 lime wedges

DIRECTIONS

1. In a small saucepan, bring 2 cups of filtered water to a simmer.
2. Add green tea bags, thyme, ginger, turmeric, honey, and apple cider vinegar.
3. Simmer gently for 5 minutes.
4. Remove from heat and let steep for another 5 minutes.
5. Strain into a pitcher or jar and cool to room temperature.
6. Refrigerate until chilled.
7. To serve: Fill a glass with ice, pour in half the tonic (about ¾ cup), top with ½ cup sparkling water, and garnish with a lime wedge.

Nutritional Facts (per serving):	
Disclaimer: *Nutritional values are estimates and may vary by ingredients and preparation.*	
Serves	2
Calories	35 kcal
Carbohydrates	9 g
Sugars	6 g
Protein	0 g
Fat	0 g
Fiber	<1 g

Lemon Ginger Tonic

Servings: 2 | Prep Time: 5 minutes

This refreshing tonic supports digestion and blood sugar regulation while delivering a boost of antioxidants and anti-inflammatory benefits. Lemon juice is high in vitamin C and may promote liver detoxification and alkalinity. Ginger offers powerful anti-inflammatory properties, aids digestion, and helps reduce nausea. Optional honey adds a touch of natural sweetness along with antimicrobial effects. Mint, used as a garnish, may help soothe the digestive tract, while cold water combined with lemon juice can support healthy blood sugar responses after meals.

INGREDIENTS

- ½ cup fresh lemon juice (from 2–3 lemons)
- 1-inch piece fresh ginger, peeled and chopped (~1 tsp grated)
- 1½ cups filtered water (still or sparkling)
- 1–2 tsp raw honey (optional; adjust to taste)
- Ice cubes
- Fresh mint leaves or lemon slices, for garnish

DIRECTIONS

1. Juice the lemons to yield about ½ cup of fresh lemon juice.
2. Peel and chop the ginger.
3. In a blender, combine lemon juice, chopped ginger, and honey (if using). Blend until smooth.
4. Strain through a fine mesh sieve into a pitcher to remove pulp.
5. Add water and stir well.
6. Serve over ice in glasses. Garnish with mint or lemon.

Nutritional Facts (per serving):	
Disclaimer: *Nutritional values are estimates and may vary by ingredients and preparation.*	
Serves	2
Calories	~22 kcal
Carbohydrates	~6 g
– Sugars	~5 g
Protein	0 g
Fat	0 g
Fiber	<0.5 g

Turmeric Ginger Honey Shots

Servings: About 7 | Prep Time: 5 minutes

This citrus ginger turmeric shot is a powerful daily tonic packed with anti-inflammatory and immune-supportive ingredients. Fresh turmeric and ginger contain compounds like curcumin and gingerol, known for reducing inflammation, supporting digestion, and enhancing immunity. The citrus fruits—lemons, limes, and tangerines—are rich in vitamin C and antioxidants, which help protect cells and support the body's natural defenses. A touch of honey adds natural sweetness and soothing properties, while black pepper enhances the absorption of curcumin, making the benefits of turmeric more bioavailable. Taken daily, this shot can support immune resilience, reduce inflammation, and promote

INGREDIENTS

- 1 whole fresh or 1 Tbsp powdered turmeric
- 1 whole fresh or 1 Tbsp powdered ginger
- Juice of 2 lemons or limes
- 2 whole tangerines, peeled
- 1 Tbsp honey
- A pinch of black pepper
- 17 oz (½ liter) water

DIRECTIONS

1. Blend all ingredients together and strain it through a rice strainer into a jar you can close.
2. Store in the fridge and take a 3.4 oz shot every day until finished.

Nutritional Facts (per serving):	
Disclaimer: *Nutritional values are estimates and may vary by ingredients and preparation.*	
Serves	7
Serving Size	1 shot (~3.4 oz / 100 ml)
Calories	~35 kcal
Protein	0.5 g
Carbohydrates	9 g
Fiber	0.5 g
Sugars	7 g (natural from citrus + honey)
Fats	0.2 g
Sodium	~1 mg
Vitamin C	~60% DV
Vitamin A	~2% DV
Calcium	~2% DV
Iron	~3% DV
Anti-inflammatory compounds	High (curcumin from turmeric, gingerol from ginger, citrus bioflavonoids)
Absorption booster	Black pepper (enhances curcumin bioavailability)

Flax Superpower Puree

Serves: About 14 | *Prep time: 5 minutes*

This flax-turmeric morning paste is a potent anti-inflammatory blend designed to support digestion, immunity, and overall wellness. Made with ground flax, turmeric, ginger, black pepper, honey, and raw apple cider vinegar, it forms a thick, nutrient-dense paste rich in antioxidants, omega-3s, and natural anti-inflammatory compounds. Taken daily by the tablespoon with water, it provides a gentle energy boost and may help reduce inflammation, support gut health, and stabilize blood sugar levels—making it a powerful addition to your morning routine.

INGREDIENTS

- 3 Tbsp ground flax
- 3 Tbsp turmeric powder
- 3 Tbsp ginger powder
- ½ Tbsp ground black pepper
- ½ cup of honey, more if needed
- 1 Tbsp apple cider vinegar with "mother"

DIRECTIONS

1. Stir all together until it forms a puree. Store in a closed jar and in the fridge.
2. Take 1 Tbsp each morning on an empty stomach with some water.

Nutritional Facts (per serving):	
Disclaimer: *Nutritional values are estimates and may vary by ingredients and preparation.*	
Serves	14
Serving Size	1 tablespoon (~20 g)
Calories	~80 kcal
Protein	0.8 g
Carbohydrates	10 g
Fiber	1.5 g
Sugars	7 g (from honey)
Fats	4 g
Saturated Fat	0.4 g
Unsaturated Fat	3.6 g
Sodium	~1 mg
Vitamin A	~0% DV
Vitamin C	~1% DV
Calcium	~2% DV
Iron	~5% DV
Magnesium	~6% DV
Potassium	~70 mg
Antioxidants	Very high (from turmeric, ginger, flaxseed, honey, and black pepper)

Lemon Olive Oil Tonic

Servings: 6 | Prep Time: 5 minutes

This is a refreshing and nutrient-packed blend designed to boost your health with every sip. As we have discussed in the book, food can act as medicine and be transformational for healing. This drink can affect changes to your skin and mood through a powerful combination of antioxidants, healthy fats, and natural sweetness. Lemons are rich in vitamin C, which supports immunity and promotes glowing skin, while olive oil contains heart-healthy monounsaturated fats that aid digestion and reduce inflammation. Organic honey not only enhances the flavor but also provides antibacterial properties and a natural energy boost. Whether you're looking to improve digestion, support your immune system, or simply enjoy a revitalizing drink, this recipe is a simple and effective addition to your wellness routine.

INGREDIENTS

- 1 whole organic lemon (thoroughly washed)
- 3 Tbsp organic honey
- 4 Tbsp organic olive oil
- 3 cups of filtered water

DIRECTIONS

1. Blend until completely liquified, about 1 minute, and strain until smooth. Drink 4 oz a day on an empty stomach. Store in the fridge and make fresh every week.

Nutritional Facts (per serving):	
Disclaimer: *Nutritional values are estimates and may vary by ingredients and preparation.*	
Serves	**6**
Serving Size	**~4 oz (½ cup / ~120 ml)**
Calories	**~120 kcal**
Protein	**0.2 g**
Carbohydrates	**10 g**
Fiber	**0.5 g**
Sugars	**8 g (from honey and lemon)**
Fats	**9 g**
Saturated Fat	**1.3 g**
Unsaturated Fat	**7.7 g**
Sodium	**~1 mg**
Vitamin A	**~0% DV**
Vitamin C	**~20% DV**
Calcium	**~1% DV**
Iron	**~2% DV**
Magnesium	**~2% DV**
Potassium	**~60 mg**
Antioxidants	**High (from lemon peel, olive oil, and honey)**

Turmeric Banana Honey Boost

Servings: 1 | Prep Time: 5 minutes

This section of health tonics is more medicinal than for pure enjoyment, but feeling good sometimes requires us to try new things we wouldn't normally think of. Food is like medicine, after all. This concoction is more for when you are starting to feel a bit under the weather. You should always consult your doctor if you feel out of the ordinary but if you know it's likely a cold that is coming on, you can try some natural remedies instead of (or in addition to) resorting to medications. Eat this mixture on an empty stomach for three to five days, and you should start feeling relief from inflammation and respiratory symptoms within just a day or two. Echinacea tea and tonic are also recommended, which you can find at most supermarkets, pharmacies, or health stores.

INGREDIENTS

- 1 banana
- ½ tsp of turmeric powder
- 1 tsp of honey
- Pinch of black pepper

DIRECTIONS

1. Mash a peeled banana with turmeric powder.
2. Add honey to enhance its anti-inflammatory benefits.
3. For extra potency, mix in a pinch of black pepper to boost turmeric's absorption.
4. Eat the entire mixture.

Nutritional Facts (per serving):	
Disclaimer: *Nutritional values are estimates and may vary by ingredients and preparation.*	
Serves	1
Serving Size	Entire mixture (~130–150 g)
Calories	~140 kcal
Protein	1.5 g
Carbohydrates	35 g
Fiber	3 g
Sugars	20 g (naturally from banana and honey)
Fats	0.5 g
Saturated Fat	0.1 g
Unsaturated Fat	0.4 g
Sodium	~1 mg
Vitamin A	~2% DV
Vitamin C	~15% DV
Calcium	~1% DV
Iron	~2% DV
Magnesium	~8% DV
Potassium	~450 mg
Antioxidants	High (from turmeric, black pepper, banana, and honey)

Super Detox Smoothie

Servings: 1–2 | *Prep Time: 5–10 minutes*

This smoothie has a detoxifying blend designed to help your body eliminate harmful heavy metals while providing essential nutrients. This smoothie combines bananas and blueberries for natural sweetness and antioxidants, while cilantro and Atlantic dulse work as powerful detoxifiers, binding to heavy metals and aiding in their removal. Spirulina, a nutrient-dense superfood, supports energy levels and immune function, while hydrating coconut water replenishes electrolytes and promotes overall wellness. Rich in vitamins, minerals, and plant-based compounds, this smoothie helps to support brain function, liver health, and cellular repair. Enjoy this refreshing and nourishing drink as part of your daily routine to gently cleanse and revitalize your body.

INGREDIENTS

- 2 bananas
- 2 cups frozen or fresh wild blueberries (or 2 oz pure wild blueberry juice or 2 Tbsp wild blueberry powder)
- 1 cup fresh cilantro (tightly packed)
- 1 tsp barley grass juice powder
- 1 tsp spirulina
- 1 Tbsp Atlantic dulse (or 2 Tbsp Atlantic dulse liquid)
- 1 orange, juiced
- ½ to 1 cup water, coconut water, or extra fresh orange juice (optional)

DIRECTIONS

1. Blend everything in a high-speed blender until smooth. If you like it a little thinner, add up to 1 cup of water. Easy to make, even easier to enjoy.

Nutritional Facts (per serving):	
Disclaimer: *Nutritional values are estimates and may vary by ingredients and preparation.*	
Serves	2
Serving Size	~1 large glass (~400–450 ml)
Calories	~170 kcal
Protein	4 g
Carbohydrates	39 g
Fiber	6 g
Sugars	21 g (naturally from fruit)
Fats	0.5 g
Saturated Fat	0 g
Unsaturated Fat	0.5 g
Sodium	~50 mg
Vitamin A	~10% DV
Vitamin C	~70% DV
Calcium	~6% DV
Iron	~15% DV
Magnesium	~18% DV
Potassium	~600 mg
Antioxidants	Very high (from wild blueberries, cilantro, orange, and spirulina)

Detoxifying Beet & Lime Tonic

Servings: 2 | *Prep Time: 5 minutes*

The tonic is a vibrant and invigorating drink that helps cleanse the body while delivering a burst of essential nutrients. While not everyone's favorite, to make up for it, beets are rich in antioxidants and nitrates, which support liver detoxification, improve circulation, and boost energy levels. Fresh lime juice adds a refreshing zing while providing vitamin C to strengthen immunity and enhance digestion. Ginger brings its natural anti-inflammatory and digestive benefits, while a touch of honey balances the flavors with its antibacterial and soothing properties. This powerful tonic is perfect for revitalizing your system, promoting glowing skin, and supporting overall wellness.

INGREDIENTS

- 1 cup chopped beets (no skin)
- 2 limes, sliced
- 1 whole ginger
- 1 cup water
- 1 Tbsp honey

DIRECTIONS

1. Blend all ingredients. Strain into a jar and store in the fridge.
2. Drink one cup every day until finished. You can add a little more honey into each serving if desired.

Nutritional Facts (per serving):	
Disclaimer: *Nutritional values are estimates and may vary by ingredients and preparation.*	
Serves	2
Serving Size	~1 cup (~240 ml)
Calories	~65 kcal
Protein	1 g
Carbohydrates	16 g
Fiber	2 g
Sugars	13 g (naturally from beets, lime, and honey)
Fats	0.2 g
Saturated Fat	0 g
Unsaturated Fat	0.2 g
Sodium	~50 mg
Vitamin A	~1% DV
Vitamin C	~40% DV
Calcium	~2% DV
Iron	~4% DV
Magnesium	~6% DV
Potassium	~300 mg
Antioxidants	Very high (from beets, lime, and ginger)

Green Juice Cleanse

Servings: 1 | Prep Time: 5 minutes

While it might be a curious combination, this is a refreshing, nutrient-dense blend designed to cleanse and energize your body. Hydrating coconut water replenishes electrolytes, while green apple and lemon juice provide a boost of vitamin C and natural sweetness. Cucumber, celery, parsley, and spinach work together to flush out toxins, support digestion, and deliver essential vitamins and minerals. Ginger adds a spicy kick with its anti-inflammatory and gut-soothing properties, while chia seeds offer fiber and omega-3s for sustained energy. This vibrant smoothie is the perfect way to nourish your body, promote digestion, and support overall wellness.

INGREDIENTS

- 1 cup coconut water
- 1 green apple, cored
- 1 inch ginger, skinned
- 4–6 inches cucumber
- 2 large celery sticks
- 2 Tbsp lemon juice
- ¼ cup chopped parsley
- 1 cup spinach
- 1 Tbsp chia seeds

DIRECTIONS

1. Blend all together and enjoy!

Nutritional Facts (per serving):	
Disclaimer: *Nutritional values are estimates and may vary by ingredients and preparation.*	
Serves	1
Serving Size	~1 large glass (~400–450 ml)
Calories	~120 kcal
Protein	3 g
Carbohydrates	22 g
Fiber	6 g
Sugars	11 g (naturally from apple, coconut water, and vegetables)
Fats	3.5 g
Saturated Fat	0.5 g
Unsaturated Fat	3 g
Sodium	~100 mg
Vitamin A	~70% DV
Vitamin C	~60% DV
Calcium	~10% DV
Iron	~15% DV
Magnesium	~18% DV
Potassium	~700 mg
Antioxidants	Very high (from spinach, parsley, ginger, lemon, and green apple)

Apple Beetroot Cinnamon Detox Water

Servings: 4 | Prep Time: 5 minutes

This water has a host ofbenefits including helping with digestion and inflammation while boosting metabolism. The apple and beetroot are loaded with antioxidants which enhance your skin's radiance and promote detoxification. Sip this nutrient-packed detox water for a refreshing way to hydrate and glow.

INGREDIENTS

- 1 small cinnamon stick
- 2 cloves
- 3–4 apple slices (thinly sliced, with skin)
- 3–4 beetroot slices (thinly sliced)
- 1 liter of water
- 2 tsp lemon juice

DIRECTIONS

1. Thinly slice the apple and beetroot for maximum flavor.
2. In a large jar or pitcher, add the cinnamon stick, cloves, apple slices, and beetroot slices.
3. Pour 1 liter of water into the jar, covering all the ingredients.
4. Let the mixture sit for at least 1–3 hours or overnight in the refrigerator to allow the flavors to develop.
5. Pour into a glass and enjoy throughout the day. Refill with water as needed for a second round.

Nutritional Facts (per serving):	
Disclaimer: *Nutritional values are estimates and may vary by ingredients and preparation.*	
Serves	4
Serving Size	~1 cup (~240 ml)
Calories	~10 kcal
Protein	0.2 g
Carbohydrates	3 g
Fiber	0.5 g (trace amounts infused)
Sugars	2 g (natural infusion from apple and beet slices)
Fats	0 g
Saturated Fat	0 g
Unsaturated Fat	0 g
Sodium	~5 mg
Vitamin A	~1% DV
Vitamin C	~6% DV (from lemon juice)
Calcium	~1% DV
Iron	~1% DV
Magnesium	~2% DV
Potassium	~50 mg
Antioxidants	High (from beet, apple peel, cinnamon, and clove infusion)

Vitamin C Wellness Shot

Servings: 12 | *Prep Time: 5 minutes*

This shot is a powerful immunity-boosting elixir packed with antioxidants and anti-inflammatory compounds. It also contains essential minerals like calcium, iron, and potassium. The green apple is naturally rich in vitamin C, helping to strengthen immunity and support glowing skin. Raw turmeric and fresh ginger work together to reduce inflammation, aid digestion, and enhance circulation, while black pepper boosts the absorption of turmeric's active compound, curcumin. A pinch of black salt adds essential minerals and enhances electrolyte balance, making this wellness shot a potent daily dose of nourishment and vitality.

INGREDIENTS

- 1 green apple
- 3-inch piece of raw turmeric
- 3-inch piece of raw ginger
- ½ tsp black pepper
- ¼ tsp black salt
- 2–2½ cups water (adjust based on desired strength)

DIRECTIONS

1. Add apple, raw turmeric, ginger, black pepper, black salt, and some water to a blender. Blend until smooth.
2. Strain the mixture through a fine mesh or muslin cloth to extract the juice. Discard the pulp.
3. Pour the juice into an airtight container and refrigerate for 3-4 days. Alternatively, pour into ice cube trays and freeze for up to a month.

Nutritional Facts (per serving):	
Disclaimer: *Nutritional values are estimates and may vary by ingredients and preparation.*	
Serves	12
Serving Size	1 shot (~2 oz / 60 ml)
Calories	~15 kcal
Protein	0.3 g
Carbohydrates	4 g
Fiber	0.5 g (mostly strained out)
Sugars	1 g (naturally from amla and ginger)
Fats	0.1 g
Saturated Fat	0 g
Unsaturated Fat	0.1 g
Sodium	~90 mg (from black salt)
Vitamin A	~1% DV
Vitamin C	~80% DV
Calcium	~2% DV
Iron	~3% DV
Magnesium	~4% DV
Potassium	~100 mg
Antioxidants	Extremely high (from amla, turmeric, ginger, and black

NOTES

Take one shot daily on an empty stomach for glowing skin and healthy hair.

Add a cube to warm water for a soothing detox drink.

Warm Almond Turmeric Milk

Servings: 1 | *Prep Time: 10 minutes*

The is a soothing, golden-hued drink packed with healing spices and nourishing ingredients. Turmeric and black pepper work together to provide powerful anti-inflammatory benefits, while saffron and cardamom add warmth and digestive support. Chopped almonds enrich the drink with healthy fats, protein, and vitamin E, promoting brain health and glowing skin. Lightly sweetened with honey, this comforting beverage is perfect for relaxation, immune support, and overall well-being. Note: Avoid dairy milk or full cream milk if you have acne-prone skin. Opt for lactose-free or plant-based alternatives for better results.

INGREDIENTS

- 1 cup plant milk of choice
- A few strands of saffron
- ¼ tsp turmeric powder
- ¼ tsp cardamom powder
- A pinch of black pepper
- 1–2 Tbsp chopped almonds
- Sweetener of choice (e.g., agave syrup, honey, or Stevia)

DIRECTIONS

1. Heat the milk in a saucepan over low to medium heat.
2. Add the saffron strands, turmeric powder, cardamom powder, and black pepper. Stir well.
3. Add the chopped almonds to the milk and let it simmer for 3–4 minutes.
4. Remove from heat and pour the milk into a glass.
5. Add your sweetener of choice and mix well.
6. Serve warm and enjoy this nourishing anti-inflammatory milk.

Nutritional Facts (per serving):	
Disclaimer: *Nutritional values are estimates and may vary by ingredients and preparation.*	
Serves	1
Serving Size	~1 cup (~240 ml)
Calories	~90 kcal
Protein	2 g
Carbohydrates	5 g
Fiber	1 g
Sugars	3 g (naturally from almonds + agave syrup)
Fats	7 g
Saturated Fat	0.5 g
Unsaturated Fat	6.5 g
Sodium	~150 mg (depends on plant milk brand)
Vitamin A	~10% DV
Vitamin C	~0% DV
Calcium	~25% DV (from fortified plant milk)
Iron	~4% DV
Magnesium	~8% DV
Potassium	~200 mg
Antioxidants	High (from saffron, turmeric, cardamom, and black pepper)

Strawberry Glow Water

Servings: 1 | Prep Time: 5 minutes

While the focus of this book is for healing, you will certainly see a difference in the way you look in addition to how you feel. Eating and drinking healthy nutrients could clear skin issues, make your skin and hair more vibrant, and glow from the inside out. This water offers a fancy drink to liven up your average water. If you have trouble with getting in your recommended water intake, this offers an exciting alternative to plain filtered water. The great aspect of this drink is it contains many vitamins inside from the fruits in addition to a bit of fiber from the chia seeds.

INGREDIENTS

- ½ chopped pineapple
- ½ sliced strawberries
- ¼ sliced beetroot
- ¼ pomegranate seeds
- ½ chopped cucumbers
- 1 Tbsp lemon juice
- A pinch of pink salt
- 1 Tbsp soaked chia seeds
- 1 liter water

DIRECTIONS

1. In a large jar, add the chopped pineapple, pomegranate sliced strawberries, beetroot, and cucumbers.
2. Squeeze in the lemon juice and sprinkle a pinch of pink salt.
3. Add the soaked chia seeds and pour in 1 liter of water.
4. Stir well, cover, and let it infuse in the refrigerator for at least 1-2 hours.
5. Enjoy chilled.

Nutritional Facts (per serving):	
Disclaimer: *Nutritional values are estimates and may vary by ingredients and preparation.*	
Serves	4
Serving Size	~1 cup (~250 ml)
Calories	~25 kcal
Protein	0.5 g
Carbohydrates	6 g
Fiber	1.5 g
Sugars	4 g (naturally from fruit)
Fats	0.5 g
Saturated Fat	0 g
Unsaturated Fat	0.5 g
Sodium	~40 mg (from pink salt)
Vitamin A	~2% DV
Vitamin C	~20% DV
Calcium	~3% DV
Iron	~2% DV
Magnesium	~4% DV
Potassium	~100 mg
Antioxidants	High (from pomegranate, beetroot, strawberries, and chia seeds)

Fennel Rose Chia Tea

Servings: 1 | *Prep Time: 5 minutes*

The tea is a fragrant and nourishing infusion that supports digestion, hydration, and relaxation. Fennel seeds and ginger powder aid in soothing the digestive system, while cardamom and rose petals provide calming and antioxidant-rich properties. Chia seeds add a dose of fiber and omega-3s, making this tea a gentle yet powerful blend for overall wellness. If you're sensitive to ginger or prone to acne, you can skip the ginger for a milder tea.

INGREDIENTS

- 1 tsp fennel seeds
- 1 tsp dried rose petals (or fresh rose petals)
- 1 tsp ginger powder (or grated ginger; avoid if prone to acne)
- 1 tsp cardamom powder
- 1 tsp soaked chia seeds
- Sweetener of choice (like honey or agave)

DIRECTIONS

1. In a pan, add water and bring it to a gentle simmer.
2. Add fennel seeds, dried rose petals, ginger powder (or grated ginger), and cardamom powder.
3. Stir well and let it simmer for 2–3 minutes to infuse the flavors.
4. Once done, strain the tea into a cup and add soaked chia seeds for an extra boost of hydration and fiber.
5. Add your sweetener and enjoy.

Nutritional Facts (per serving):	
Disclaimer: *Nutritional values are estimates and may vary by ingredients and preparation.*	
Serves	1
Serving Size	~1 cup (~250 ml)
Calories	~30 kcal
Protein	0.5 g
Carbohydrates	6 g
Fiber	2 g (mostly from chia seeds)
Sugars	3–4 g (depends on sweetener and amount used)
Fats	1.5 g
Saturated Fat	0.1 g
Unsaturated Fat	1.4 g
Sodium	~5 mg
Vitamin A	~1% DV
Vitamin C	~2% DV
Calcium	~5% DV
Iron	~6% DV
Magnesium	~6% DV
Potassium	~80 mg
Antioxidants	High (from rose petals, fennel, cardamom, ginger)

Healing Citrus Cubes

Servings: 12 cubes / about 1 oz per cube | *Prep Time: 5 minutes*

This tonic is a vibrant and revitalizing blend designed to support overall health and wellness. Lemons and oranges provide a powerful dose of vitamin C and antioxidants, while turmeric, ginger, and cinnamon work together to reduce inflammation and aid digestion. Black pepper enhances the absorption of turmeric's curcumin, making this tonic a potent immunity booster and energizing addition to your daily routine.

INGREDIENTS

- 2 lemons, peeled
- 2 oranges, peeled
- 250g (9-10 oz) turmeric, washed
- 250g (9-10 oz) ginger, washed
- Pinch of pepper

DIRECTIONS

1. Add everything in a juicer and juice, or a blender and blend/strain.
2. Pour into an ice cube tray and freeze overnight.
3. Enjoy each cube by popping it into some hot water so it melts into a tea. Or by adding it to a lemonade for a cooler drink.

Nutritional Facts (per serving):	
Disclaimer: *Nutritional values are estimates and may vary by ingredients and preparation.*	
Serves	12
Serving Size	1 cube (~2–2.5 oz / 60–75 ml)
Calories	~25 kcal
Protein	0.5 g
Carbohydrates	6 g
Fiber	1 g
Sugars	3 g (naturally from lemon and orange)
Fats	0.3 g
Saturated Fat	0 g
Unsaturated Fat	0.3 g
Sodium	~2 mg
Vitamin A	~1% DV
Vitamin C	~20% DV
Calcium	~2% DV
Iron	~3% DV
Magnesium	~5% DV
Potassium	~110 mg
Antioxidants	Very high (from turmeric, ginger, citrus, and black pepper)

Blueberry Antioxidant Smoothie

Servings: 1 smoothie **|** *Prep Time: 5 minutes*

This smoothie is a hydrating and antioxidant-rich blend that nourishes the body while supporting digestion and immunity. Coconut water replenishes electrolytes, while blueberries and lemon provide a boost of vitamin C and powerful antioxidants to combat inflammation. Avocado adds healthy fats for sustained energy, and turmeric with black pepper enhances anti-inflammatory benefits, making this smoothie a perfect choice for daily wellness.

INGREDIENTS

- 1 cup coconut water
- ½ frozen blueberries
- 1 small cube of ginger, peeled
- Juice of ½ lemon
- ½ avocado
- 1 tsp turmeric
- Pinch of black pepper

DIRECTIONS

1. Blend together and enjoy!

Nutritional Facts (per serving):	
Disclaimer: *Nutritional values are estimates and may vary by ingredients and preparation.*	
Serves	1
Serving Size	~1 smoothie (~300–350 ml)
Calories	~180 kcal
Protein	2 g
Carbohydrates	18 g
Fiber	6 g
Sugars	9 g (naturally from blueberries, lemon, and coconut water)
Fats	12 g
Saturated Fat	2.5 g
Unsaturated Fat	9.5 g
Sodium	~85 mg
Vitamin A	~6% DV
Vitamin C	~35% DV
Calcium	~4% DV
Iron	~6% DV
Magnesium	~12% DV
Potassium	~500 mg
Antioxidants	Very high (from blueberries, turmeric, ginger, lemon, and avocado)

Turmeric Ginger Honey Tea

Servings: 4 | *Prep Time: 10 minutes*

This recipe is very simple with minimal effort. One thing to note is, for your plant milk, the thicker the consistency the better for frothing. So something like Oatly or any type of Barista Edition plant milk would be best. Otherwise, it is too thin and won't froth properly. The frothy milk is of course optional, but makes it more enjoyable. You can also add it as-is for a tea-like consistency. Lastly, you probably have a small mesh tea ball infuser at home without knowing it. This is the little ball with holes in it where you can add tea leaves. If you don't have it, you can simply add the turmeric and ginger freely and strain it out after.

INGREDIENTS

- 1 tsp fresh ginger
- 1 tsp fresh turmeric
- Tea of choice
- Honey (optional)
- Stainless steel tea ball infuser

DIRECTIONS

1. Grate the ginger and turmeric until you get about 1 tsp each. Add to your tea infuser.
2. Pour in boiling water and let steep for at least 5–10 minutes. Add honey.
3. Remove the infuser and enjoy your tea!

Nutritional Facts (per serving):	
Disclaimer: *Nutritional values are estimates and may vary by ingredients and preparation.*	
Serves	1
Serving Size	~1 cup brewed tea (~240 ml) honey not included
Calories	~5 kcal
Protein	0.2 g
Carbohydrates	1 g
Fiber	0.3 g (minimal in strained tea)
Sugars	0 g
Fats	0 g
Saturated Fat	0 g
Unsaturated Fat	0 g
Sodium	~1 mg
Vitamin A	~0% DV
Vitamin C	~1% DV
Calcium	~1% DV
Iron	~1% DV
Magnesium	~2% DV
Potassium	~40 mg
Antioxidants	Very high (from fresh ginger and turmeric)

Jar of Ginger Wellness Tea

Servings: About 12 shots | *Prep Time: 10 minutes*

This is a soothing and invigorating blend that promotes digestion and boosts immunity with every sip. Ginger and turmeric work together to reduce inflammation and support joint health, while a splash of lemon provides vitamin C to strengthen your immune system. The addition of black pepper enhances turmeric's absorption, making this tea a powerful and refreshing remedy for overall wellness. You can also freeze this juice in an ice cube tray and to consume, pour some hot water over one cube whenever you are feeling a cold coming on.

INGREDIENTS

- 2 cups fresh organic ginger root, washed
- 3–4 whole organic lemons, washed with the two ends cut off
- 2–3 cups filtered water
- 1–2 Tbsp of turmeric powder (or whole turmeric root)
- 1–2 Tbsp of honey (manuka preferred)
- Pinch of black pepper

DIRECTIONS

1. Blend the ginger, lemons, and water in a blender.
2. Strain into a large jar. Toss the pulp.
3. Pour the strained juice back in the blender and add turmeric powder, pepper, and honey. Blend until combined.
4. Store in the fridge for about a week. To consume, I recommend a small shot every day with some hot water added in to make a tea and reduce the intensity of ginger.

Nutritional Facts (per serving):	
Disclaimer: *Nutritional values are estimates and may vary by ingredients and preparation.*	
Serves	12
Serving Size	~2 oz (~60 ml)
Calories	~25 kcal
Protein	0.3 g
Carbohydrates	6 g
Fiber	~0.3 g (mostly strained out)
Sugars	3.5 g (naturally from lemon + honey)
Fats	0.1 g
Saturated Fat	0 g
Unsaturated Fat	0.1 g
Sodium	~1 mg
Vitamin A	~1% DV
Vitamin C	~18% DV
Calcium	~1% DV
Iron	~2% DV
Magnesium	~2% DV
Potassium	~70 mg
Antioxidants	Very high (from ginger, turmeric, lemon, and black pepper)

Sweet Turmeric Latte

Servings: 1–2 | Prep Time: 5 minutes

This latte is a creamy and invigorating drink that combines the boldness of black coffee with the anti-inflammatory benefits of turmeric. Sweetened with honey, this latte offers a natural energy boost while providing antioxidants and essential vitamins from turmeric and coconut milk. The healthy fats in coconut milk support brain function and promote a sense of calm, making this latte a perfect balance of flavor and nourishment.

INGREDIENTS

- ½ cup strongly brewed black coffee
- 2 tsp turmeric powder
- 1 Tbsp honey
- 1 cup coconut milk, steamed/frothed

DIRECTIONS

1. Make your coffee. Add the steamed milk to the hot coffee, then stir in the turmeric powder and honey.

Nutritional Facts (per serving):	
Disclaimer: *Nutritional values are estimates and may vary by ingredients and preparation.*	
Serves	1
Serving Size	~1 mug (~10–12 oz)
Calories	~160 kcal
Protein	6 g
Carbohydrates	19 g
Fiber	0 g
Sugars	17 g (from honey and milk)
Fats	7 g
Saturated Fat	4.5 g
Unsaturated Fat	2.5 g
Sodium	~80 mg
Vitamin A	~10% DV
Vitamin C	~1% DV
Calcium	~20% DV
Iron	~2% DV
Magnesium	~6% DV
Potassium	~250 mg
Antioxidants	High (from turmeric, coffee, and honey)

Matcha Collagen Smoothie

Servings: 1 | Prep Time: 5 minutes

This Matcha Collagen Smoothie is a vibrant and energizing drink that combines the rich antioxidants of matcha with the nourishing benefits of collagen. Matcha boosts metabolism and enhances focus, while the banana provides natural sweetness and potassium for muscle function. Grass-fed milk offers healthy fats and protein, supporting bone health and skin elasticity, making this smoothie a perfect blend for both vitality and beauty.

INGREDIENTS

- 2 tsp matcha powder
- 1 cup grass-fed milk or plant milk
- ½ frozen banana
- 1 scoop collagen powder of choice, in vanilla or unflavored

DIRECTIONS

1. Stir matcha powder into the milk, then blend all ingredients together.

Nutritional Facts (per serving):	
Disclaimer: *Nutritional values are estimates and may vary by ingredients and preparation.*	
Serves	1
Serving Size	~1 glass (~10–12 oz / 300–350 ml) using grass fed milk
Calories	~210 kcal
Protein	14 g
Carbohydrates	17 g
Fiber	2 g
Sugars	10 g (naturally from banana and milk)
Fats	9 g
Saturated Fat	5 g
Unsaturated Fat	4 g
Sodium	~100 mg
Vitamin A	~10% DV
Vitamin C	~8% DV
Calcium	~30% DV
Iron	~4% DV
Magnesium	~10% DV
Potassium	~400 mg
Antioxidants	High (from matcha and banana)

Ginger Lemonade

Servings: 1–2 | *Prep Time: 5 minutes*

Lemonade is one of my favorite refreshing drinks. However, store-purchased drinks often are made from concentrate and filled with sugar. Making it at home allows you to control the sugar and keep the antioxidant benefits of using real lemons. I recommend preparing this in a jar at the start of the week (don't add ice cubes until serving it) and having it to accompany your meals. It's sweet and familiar, with the cleansing effect of natural lemons. It also contains ginger to provide anti-inflammatory benefits as well.

INGREDIENTS

- 1-inch piece fresh ginger, peeled and grated
- ½ cup lemon juice
- 2 Tbsp honey
- 2 cups water
- 1 cup ice cubes

DIRECTIONS

1. Add lemon juice, water, and ice cubes to a glass, then mix in the grated ginger and honey.

Nutritional Facts (per serving):	
Disclaimer: *Nutritional values are estimates and may vary by ingredients and preparation.*	
Serves	2
Serving Size	~1 cup (~240 ml)
Calories	~45 kcal
Protein	0.2 g
Carbohydrates	12 g
Fiber	~0.3 g
Sugars	10 g (from honey and lemon)
Fats	0 g
Saturated Fat	0 g
Unsaturated Fat	0 g
Sodium	~1 mg
Vitamin A	~0% DV
Vitamin C	~30% DV
Calcium	~1% DV
Iron	~1% DV
Magnesium	~2% DV
Potassium	~100 mg
Antioxidants	High (from fresh ginger and lemon juice)

Berry Mint Tea

Servings: 1 jar | *Prep Time: 10 minutes*

Mint has become one of my favorite herbs in the last few years not only because of its refreshing taste but because of its soothing digestive benefits. If you have never tried Moroccan mint tea, you are missing out on one of the great joys of life. Even if you can't make it to Morocco, you can likely find it in many North African or Arab restaurants in your area, or you can make it at home. This is not a recipe for Moroccan tea, however, but an experiment for a fruity and tummy-soothing tea. And of course, I have included mint in this recipe. The combined benefits of mint with ginger and cinnamon, balanced with the sweet berries, offers a unique blend you probably haven't tried yet. Let's not forget, it is comforting and tastes delicious.

INGREDIENTS

- ¾ cup frozen wild blueberries or raspberries
- 2 slices of lemon
- Handful of fresh mint leaves
- 1 inch ginger, peeled and sliced
- 2 cinnamon sticks
- 4–6 cups boiling water

DIRECTIONS

1. Combine all in a tea jug and steep for 5–10 minutes.

Nutritional Facts (per serving):	
Disclaimer: *Nutritional values are estimates and may vary by ingredients and preparation.*	
Serves	4
Serving Size	~1½ cups (~350 ml)
Calories	~10 kcal
Protein	0.1 g
Carbohydrates	3 g
Fiber	0.5 g
Sugars	2 g (naturally from blueberries and lemon)
Fats	0 g
Saturated Fat	0 g
Unsaturated Fat	0 g
Sodium	~1 mg
Vitamin A	~2% DV
Vitamin C	~10% DV
Calcium	~1% DV
Iron	~1% DV
Magnesium	~2% DV
Potassium	~60 mg
Antioxidants	Very high (from blueberries, cinnamon, ginger, and mint)

Carrot Apple Orange Juice

Servings: 4 | Prep Time: 5 minutes

This juice contains all the orange things. Luckily, they pair well together in the taste department as well. You may already know that carrots are good for the skin and eyes. However, carrot juice is also excellent for helping remove old bile from the liver, which gives a cleansing effect to your body. Studies have also shown carrot juice to boost brain health, improve memory, and even lower cognitive stress in the brain. Apples and oranges also contain similar inflammation-reducing vitamins and fiber. They are both also great for your immune system during your healing journey.

INGREDIENTS

- 2 apples
- 2 oranges
- 8–12 carrots

DIRECTIONS

1. Juice or blend together and strain.

Nutritional Facts (per serving):	
Disclaimer: *Nutritional values are estimates and may vary by ingredients and preparation.*	
Serves	4
Serving Size	~1 cup (~240–250 ml)
Calories	~110 kcal
Protein	1.5 g
Carbohydrates	26 g
Fiber	2 g (less if strained)
Sugars	20 g (naturally from fruit and carrots)
Fats	0.3 g
Saturated Fat	0 g
Unsaturated Fat	0.3 g
Sodium	~70 mg
Vitamin A	~350% DV
Vitamin C	~80% DV
Calcium	~4% DV
Iron	~3% DV
Magnesium	~6% DV
Potassium	~450 mg
Antioxidants	Very high (from carrots, oranges, and apples)

Anti-Inflammatory Mango Smoothie

Servings: 1 **|** *Prep Time: 5 minutes*

Mango does not get enough attention in my opinion, as it is one of the fruits that contains the most sugar. However, the trade off for its delicious sweetness is that it also contains so many vitamins, as well as minerals like potassium, magnesium, and folate. It's also great for digestion, eye, and bone health. So, like anything, it's all about balance. Enjoy this smoothie whenever you want a fresh and sweet treat. The creamy yogurt and banana make this almost a dessert.

INGREDIENTS

- 1 cup frozen mango
- 1 medium banana
- ½ cup plant milk
- ½ cup Greek yogurt, mango flavored preferred
- 1 Tbsp lemon juice
- 2 tsp grated fresh turmeric or ¾ tsp ground turmeric
- ¼ tsp cardamom
- ⅛ tsp grated fresh ginger or ⅛ tsp ground ginger (optional)
- Unsweetened shredded coconut (optional)

DIRECTIONS

1. Blend all together and pour it into a glass. Garnish with coconut if desired.

Nutritional Facts (per serving):	
Disclaimer: *Nutritional values are estimates and may vary by ingredients and preparation.*	
Serves	1
Serving Size	~1 smoothie (~350–400 ml)
Calories	~260 kcal
Protein	8 g
Carbohydrates	44 g
Fiber	4 g
Sugars	31 g (naturally from fruit and yogurt)
Fats	5 g
Saturated Fat	2.5 g
Unsaturated Fat	2.5 g
Sodium	~70 mg
Vitamin A	~35% DV
Vitamin C	~70% DV
Calcium	~20% DV
Iron	~6% DV
Magnesium	~10% DV
Potassium	~600 mg
Antioxidants	High (from turmeric, mango, banana, ginger, and lemon)

Tropical Tummy Smoothie

Servings: 1–2 | *Prep Time: 5 minutes*

Pineapple is one of the best fruits for digestion as it naturally contains bromelain, an important digestive enzyme. It also contains a variety of vitamins, antioxidants, and minerals all while tasting delicious. It is one of my favorite fruits. Ginger is an anti-inflammatory and a powerful painkiller for joint, muscle, or nerve pain. I try to add ginger to my smoothies every day for this reason. Frozen fruits are preferred for this recipe to get that cold creamy texture. Just make sure to add a bit more water or plant milk so it blends easily. If you use fresh fruit, however, make sure to add some ice cubes to get the smoothie texture.

INGREDIENTS

- 1 banana
- 2 cups chopped pineapple
- 2 cups chopped mango
- 1 inch piece peeled ginger
- 1 cup water or coconut water

DIRECTIONS

1. Blend together and enjoy fresh right away (smoothies don't store well).

Nutritional Facts (per serving):	
Disclaimer: *Nutritional values are estimates and may vary by ingredients and preparation.*	
Serves	2
Serving Size	~1½ cups (~350–400 ml)
Calories	~170 kcal
Protein	2 g
Carbohydrates	43 g
Fiber	4 g
Sugars	34 g (naturally from fruit)
Fats	0.5 g
Saturated Fat	0 g
Unsaturated Fat	0.5 g
Sodium	~10 mg
Vitamin A	~20% DV
Vitamin C	~100% DV
Calcium	~3% DV
Iron	~4% DV
Magnesium	~10% DV
Potassium	~500 mg
Antioxidants	Very high (from pineapple, mango, banana, and ginger)

Chia Flax Fiber Drink

Servings: 1 | Prep Time: 15 minutes

If you need to get things moving in your digestion, this drink is up to the task. Chia seeds aid digestion and support gut health, and flax seeds are rich in nutrients and antioxidants. They can heal a variety of ailments and inflammation. Both are a great source of fiber as well. I recommend drinking this in the morning to allow time for your body to flush itself out.

INGREDIENTS

- 2 tsp of chia seeds
- 2 tsp of flax seeds
- 1 cup water
- 1 cup plant milk
- 1 tsp sweetener of choice

DIRECTIONS

1. Add chia seeds and black seeds to a cup of water.
2. Let them soak for 10 minutes. It will produce a gel-like texture.
3. After soaking, strain the seeds and blend them with plant milk and sweeter for a creamy consistency.

Nutritional Facts (per serving):	
Disclaimer: *Nutritional values are estimates and may vary by ingredients and preparation.*	
Serves	1
Serving Size	~1½ cups (~350 ml)
Calories	~130 kcal
Protein	4 g
Carbohydrates	6 g
Fiber	5 g
Sugars	1–2 g (depending on sweetener used)
Fats	10 g
Saturated Fat	1 g
Unsaturated Fat	9 g
Sodium	~100 mg (varies by plant milk)
Vitamin A	~10% DV
Vitamin C	~0% DV
Calcium	~20% DV (from fortified plant milk)
Iron	~8% DV
Magnesium	~15% DV
Potassium	~150 mg
Antioxidants	High (from black seeds and chia seeds)

Beet Celery Apple Juice

Servings: 2 | Prep Time: 5 minutes

While the idea of this juice is probably not the most enticing you have ever heard, the benefits are worth the strange combination. This is a liver-cleansing juice packed with nutrients that will help detoxify your liver and boost your energy. Beets are rich in vitamin C and betaine, the latter which can reduce fat buildup in the liver and promote detoxification. Beets could also assist in lowering your blood pressure and act as a prebiotic for gut health. Celery is full of potassium for your muscle and organ functions and antioxidants to protect against oxidative stress. It also stimulates liver enzymes, helping flush out toxins from your system. Oranges and apples contain vitamin C and malic acid, which aids in removing heavy metals from your body, creating the perfect synergy for a deep cleanse. Like many juices, you don't usually go in for the taste but for the numerous benefits they provide.

INGREDIENTS

- 1 beetroot, peeled and chopped
- 2 celery sticks
- 1 apple, chopped
- Juice of 1 orange
- 1 cup water

DIRECTIONS

1. Peel and chop your fruits. Juice your orange.
2. Blend together and enjoy.

Nutritional Facts (per serving):	
Disclaimer: *Nutritional values are estimates and may vary by ingredients and preparation.*	
Serves	2
Serving Size	~1 cup (~240–250 ml)
Calories	~80 kcal
Protein	1 g
Carbohydrates	20 g
Fiber	3 g
Sugars	15 g (naturally from apple, beet, and orange)
Fats	0.3 g
Saturated Fat	0 g
Unsaturated Fat	0.3 g
Sodium	~50 mg
Vitamin A	~2% DV
Vitamin C	~45% DV
Calcium	~2% DV
Iron	~4% DV
Magnesium	~6% DV
Potassium	~350 mg
Antioxidants	Very high (from beetroot, apple, orange juice, and celery)

Drink the Rainbow Smoothie

Prep Time: 5 minutes | *Serves: 1*

The shining quality about smoothies is you can pack tons of nutrients into one serving. You can customize them however you like, too, which is how I discovered this recipe. Through trial and error, this one served the perfect balance of creamy, thick but still smooth, sweet but not overpowering, and refreshing but also comforting. And never fear, you cannot even taste the greens inside as they are disguised by the natural sweetness of the fruit. If you don't have coconut water, you can also use plant-based milk, but it's preferable to use coconut water due to the extra electrolytes it will provide.

INGREDIENTS

- ½ cup frozen banana
- 3 frozen strawberries
- ¼ cup frozen blueberries
- ½ clementine, peeled
- 1 cup of spinach
- 1½ cups of coconut water
- 1 scoop of vanilla or flavorless protein powder (optional)

DIRECTIONS

1. Pour 1 cup of coconut water into your blender (save the last half cup).
2. Add your frozen fruit, powder, and spinach.
3. Top it off with the remaining half cup of coconut water and blend!

Nutritional Facts (per serving):	
Disclaimer: *Nutritional values are estimates and may vary by ingredients and preparation.*	
Serves	1
Serving Size	~1 smoothie (~400–450 ml) with protein powder
Calories	~220 kcal
Protein	21 g
Carbohydrates	22 g
Fiber	5 g
Sugars	14 g (naturally from fruit and coconut water)
Fats	2 g
Saturated Fat	0.5 g
Unsaturated Fat	1.5 g
Sodium	~160 mg
Vitamin A	~50% DV
Vitamin C	~90% DV
Calcium	~15% DV
Iron	~10% DV
Magnesium	~15% DV
Potassium	~700 mg
Antioxidants	High (from spinach, berries, and citrus)

CONCLUSION

As we reach the end of this journey together, I find myself reflecting on the remarkable path that brought this book into being. It began with that seemingly ordinary day playing catch with my son—the moment when my mallet finger injury led me down an unexpected path of discovering food's profound healing power. What started as my personal quest to avoid surgery grew into something much larger: a deep understanding of how nutrition can transform the surgical experience for countless patients.

Throughout these pages, we've explored the intricate dance between food and healing that has evolved over billions of years. We've delved into the building blocks of macronutrients and the catalytic power of micronutrients. We've examined the challenges of modern food systems and how to navigate them. We've created roadmaps for pre-surgery preparation, post-operative recovery, and long-term wellness. All of these elements form a comprehensive approach to supporting your body's natural healing wisdom.

Little did I know when writing the final chapters of this book that the universe would soon present me with the ultimate test of these principles. As I shared in the introduction, just as I was completing this manuscript, I discovered through routine screening that I had a genetic heart condition requiring open heart surgery. Suddenly, the researcher became the research subject; the doctor became the patient.

Facing open heart surgery was undoubtedly one of the most challenging experiences of my life. The fear and uncertainty that accompany such a diagnosis are profound, even for someone who has spent decades in operating rooms. Yet amid this challenge, I found myself extraordinarily well-equipped. The very protocols I had developed for this book became my personal healing blueprint.

In the weeks leading up to my surgery, I meticulously followed the nutritional preparation guidelines outlined in Chapter 6. I increased my protein intake, focused on anti-inflammatory foods, optimized my vitamin and mineral levels, and implemented the carbohydrate loading strategy. My surgical team supported my preparation efforts.

Following surgery, I continued to apply these principles with unwavering dedication. Despite the significance of open heart surgery, I was discharged from the hospital after only four days—well ahead of the typical timeline. As I write these words six weeks post-surgery, my recovery continues to progress remarkably well. My energy has returned more quickly than expected, my wound has healed beautifully, and I've been able to gradually resume normal activities with surprising ease.

This experience has transformed what was already a deeply researched book into something more: a lived testimony to the power of nutritional healing. Every recommendation, every strategy, and every recipe has been filtered not just through scientific research and clinical experience, but through my own healing journey.

I share this not to boast, but to offer hope and empowerment. If these approaches could support my recovery from one of medicine's most significant surgical procedures, imagine what they might do for your healing journey.

I hope this guide has helped you understand the power you hold through your food choices. Your body has an incredible capacity for healing—a wisdom refined over billions of years of evolution. Your role is to support that wisdom with mindful, nurturing nutrition. Each meal you consume is not just sustenance; it's information for your cells, instructions for your body's healing processes, and fuel for your recovery.

Recovery, whether from a minor procedure or major surgery, is rarely a perfectly linear process. There will likely be challenges along the way—perhaps fatigue, pain, or moments of discouragement. In these times, remember that healing takes patience. Trust the process, follow the guidelines that resonate with your situation, and listen to your body's signals.

If your journey takes unexpected turns, as mine did, remember that you are resilient. Your body contains the accumulated wisdom of countless generations that have faced challenges and survived. Nurture this inherent capacity with good nutrition, positive mindset, and patience.

Thank you for allowing me to be part of your healing journey. If you're interested in staying connected and learning more about nutritional approaches to healing, you can find me at: @kamiparsamd on Instagram, Facebook, YouTube, X, and TikTok.

Remember, every meal is an opportunity to support your body's natural healing wisdom. Choose wisely, and trust in the process.

Wishing you health, healing, and wholeness on your journey.

With love & kindness,
Kami Parsa, MD

SOURCES

Chapters 1–3

Pre and Post Surgery Nutrition and Lifestyle Strategies to Optimize your Recovery - Canadian Digestive Health Foundation (cdhf ca)

Pre- and Post-Surgical Nutrition for Preservation of Muscle Mass, Strength, and Functionality Following Orthopedic Surgery - PMC (nih.gov)

"Diet approach before and after bariatric surgery" PMC (nih.gov)

Gillis. "Pre-operative nutrition and the elective surgical patient: why, how and what?" (2019) Anaesthesia - Wiley Online Library.

Hirsch, Katie R., Robert R. Wolfe and Arny A. Ferrando. "Pre- and Post-Surgical Nutrition for Preservation of Muscle Mass, Strength, and Functionality Following Orthopedic Surgery." Nutrients 13 (2021). https://www.semanticscholar.org/paper/Pre-and-Post-Surgical-Nutrition-for-Preservation-of-Hirsch-Wolfe/6bffa80cefcfa937dcd88592bae21af8c6e80313 ; https://www.ncbi.nlm.nih.gov/pmc/articles/PMC8156786/

Dr. Nancy R. Rodriguez. "The Rehabilitative Role of Protein: Protein Intake and Recovery of Muscle Mass, Strength, and Function" (31 October 2021). https://www.mdpi.com/journal/nutrients/special_issues/protein-muscle

Shoulder Doc. "Post-surgery Nutrition." https://www.shoulderdoc.co.uk/news/view/1441

Martínez Steele, E., et al. "Ultra-processed foods and added sugars in the US diet: evidence from a nationally representative cross-sectional study." BMJ Open, 2016.

Monteiro, C. A., et al. "Dietary guidelines to nourish humanity and the planet in the twenty-first century. A blueprint from Brazil." Public Health Nutrition, 2015.

Lawrence, M. A., & Baker, P. I. "Ultra-processed food and adverse health outcomes." BMJ, 2019.

Moubarac, J.-C., et al. "Consumption of ultra-processed foods and likely impact on human health. Evidence from the literature." Public Health Nutrition, 2018.

Fardet, A., "Minimally processed foods are more satiating and less hyperglycemic than ultra-processed foods." Food & Function, 2016.

Tavares, L. F., et al. "Dietary patterns and ultra-processed foods: a systematic review." Public Health Nutrition, 2017.

The importance of nutrition in wound management: new evidence from the past decade. Cambridge Media Journals.

Chapter 5

Black, D. S., O'Reilly, G. A., Olmstead, R., Breen, E. C., & Irwin, M. R. (2015). Mindfulness meditation and improvement in sleep quality and daytime impairment among older adults with sleep disturbances. JAMA Internal Medicine, 175(4), 494–501.

Black, D. S., & Slavich, G. M. (2016). Mindfulness meditation and the immune system: A systematic review of randomized controlled trials. Annals of the New York Academy of Sciences, 1373(1), 13–24.

Brook, R. D., et al. (2013). Beyond medications and diet: Alternative approaches to lowering blood pressure. Hypertension, 61(6), 1360–1383.

Buric, I., et al. (2017). What is the molecular signature of mind–body interventions? A systematic review of gene expression changes induced by meditation and related practices. Frontiers in Immunology, 8, 670.

Cherkin, D. C., et al. (2016). Effect of mindfulness-based stress reduction vs cognitive behavioral therapy or usual care on back pain and functional limitations. JAMA, 315(12), 1240–1249.

Creswell, J. D., et al. (2012). Mindfulness-based stress reduction training reduces loneliness and pro-inflammatory gene expression in older adults. Brain, Behavior, and Immunity, 26(7), 1095–1101.

Davidson, R. J., et al. (2003). Alterations in brain and immune function produced by mindfulness meditation. Psychosomatic Medicine, 65(4), 564–570.

Halpin, L. S., Speir, A. M., Capo, G., & Barnett, S. D. (2002). Guided imagery in patients undergoing CABG: A randomized, placebo-controlled pilot study. American Journal of Critical Care, 11(6), 582–588.

Kwekkeboom, K. L., Cherwin, C. H., Lee, J. W., & Wanta, B. (2010). Guided imagery for cancer pain and anxiety: A randomized clinical trial. Oncology Nursing Forum, 37(3), 397–405.

Monti, D. A., et al. (2006). A randomized, controlled trial of mindfulness-based art therapy (MBAT) for women with cancer. Psycho-Oncology, 15(5), 363–373.

Posadzki, P., et al. (2012). Guided imagery for non-musculoskeletal pain: A systematic review. The Journal of Alternative and Complementary Medicine, 18(6), 516–532.

Schneider, R. H., et al. (2012). Stress reduction in the secondary prevention of cardiovascular disease. Circulation: Cardiovascular Quality and Outcomes, 5(6), 750–758.

Zeidan, F., et al. (2011). Brain mechanisms supporting the modulation of pain by mindfulness meditation. The Journal of Neuroscience, 31(14), 5540–5548.

Chapter 6

University Of Texas At Austin (December 3, 2004). *Science Daily*. "Study Suggests Nutrient Decline In Garden Crops Over Past 50 Years." https://www.sciencedaily.com/releases/2004/12/041203100522.htm

Zulfiqar, Usman, et al. (16 February 2024). Volume 24, article number 34, (2024). *Springer Nature Link*. "Genetic biofortification: advancing crop nutrition to tackle hidden hunger." https://www.sciencedaily.com/releases/2004/12/041203100522.htm

Nordlee, Julie A. et al. (March 14, 1996). *The New England Journal of Medicine*. "Identification of a Brazil-Nut Allergen in Transgenic Soybeans." Volume 334 No. 11. https://www.nejm.org/doi/full/10.1056/NEJM199603143341103

Wischmeyer, P. E., et al. (2018). *Anesthesia & Analgesia*, 126(6), 1883-1895. Indexed at: "nearly 50% of hospitalized patients are malnourished or at risk of malnutrition before surgery" [1].

Braga, M., et al. (2002) *Surgery*, 132(5), 805-814. Indexed at: "preoperative immunonutrition reduced postoperative infectious complications by 39%" [2].

Burden, S., et al. (2012) *Cochrane Database of Systematic Reviews*, (11). Indexed at: "perioperative nutritional support significantly reduced the risk of surgical site infections" [3].

Ferrando, A. A., et al. (2013) *Journal of Parenteral and Enteral Nutrition*, 37(5_suppl), 5S-20S. Indexed at: “preoperative nutritional optimization led to reduced length of hospital stay” [4].

Wischmeyer, P. E. (2018) *Critical Care Clinics*, 34(1), 107-125. Indexed at: “Recommended intake: Current guidelines suggest 1.2–2.0 g/kg/day of protein for surgical patients” [5].

Katsanos, C. S., et al. (2006) *American Journal of Physiology-Endocrinology and Metabolism*, 291(2), E381-E387. Indexed at: Not specifically indexed in the transcript.

Bikker, A., et al. (2016) *Clinical Nutrition ESPEN*, 15, 118-122. Indexed at: Not specifically indexed in the transcript.

Ljungqvist, O. (2009) *Best Practice & Research Clinical Anaesthesiology*, 23(4), 401-409. Indexed at: “Preoperative carbohydrate loading” [8].

Nygren, J., et al. (2001) *Clinical Nutrition*, 20(1), 51-56. Indexed at: “Preoperative oral carbohydrate administration reduces postoperative insulin resistance” [9].

Practice Guidelines for Preoperative Fasting. (2017) *Anesthesiology*, 126(3), 376-393. Indexed at: “Follow your doctor’s instructions on when to stop drinking before surgery” [10].

Holte, K., & Kehlet, H. (2002) *Acta Anaesthesiologica Scandinavica*, 46(9), 1089-1093. Indexed at: “Proper hydration is crucial for optimal surgical outcomes” [11].

Suresh, S., & Sardesai, A. (2017) *BJA Education*, 17(9), 307-313. Indexed at: “Preoperative carbohydrate loading can decrease insulin resistance” [Suresh & Sardesai, 2017].

Smith, M. D., et al. (2017) *British Journal of Surgery*, 104(3), 187-197. Indexed at: "Preoperative carbohydrate administration decreased postoperative length of stay" [Smith et al., 2017].

Zhao, J., et al. (2021) *Journal of Clinical Anesthesia*, 68, 110084. Indexed at: Not specifically indexed in the transcript.

Dreno, B., et al. (2019). "Vitamin C in the healing process." *Journal of Dermatological Science*, 94(1), 40-43.

Thevi, R., et al. (2023). "Vitamin C supplementation and wound healing: A systematic review." *Clinical Nutrition*, 42(2), 223-231.

Li, Y., et al. (2016). "The role of vitamin C in tissue repair and inflammation reduction in dental surgery patients." *Journal of Periodontology*, 87(8), 884-891.

Arnljots, R., et al. (2017). "Vitamin D deficiency and its association with hip fracture recovery." *Osteoporosis International*, 28(3), 1047-1054.

Bolland, M. J., et al. (2018). "Vitamin D and musculoskeletal health." *The Lancet Diabetes & Endocrinology*, 6(11), 847-858.

Bogunovic, L., et al. (2010). "Vitamin D deficiency in orthopedic surgery patients." *The Journal of Bone and Joint Surgery*, 92(2), 297-303.

Saghiri, M. A., et al. (2015). "The role of vitamin A in wound healing." *Journal of Investigative Dermatology*, 135(5), 1285-1293.

Shamsi, M., et al. (2017). "Vitamin A and its role in collagen formation." *Clinical Nutrition Research*, 6(3), 147-157.

Hunt, T. K., et al. (2012). "Vitamin A and pressure ulcer healing." *Advances in Wound Care*, 1(1), 20-23.

Zinc: 24. Lansdown, A. B. G., et al. (2007). “Zinc in wound healing: Theoretical, experimental, and clinical aspects.” *Wound Repair and Regeneration*, 15(1), 2-16.

Lin, P. H., et al. (2017). “Zinc and its role in DNA synthesis and cell proliferation.” *Nutrition Research*, 37, 1-9.

Agren, M. S., et al. (2007). “Zinc oxide improves wound healing in chronic leg ulcers.” *The British Journal of Dermatology*, 156(5), 826-832.

Avery, J. C., & Hoffmann, P. R. (2018). “The essential role of selenium in immune function.” *Journal of Nutritional Biochemistry*, 55, 1-14.

Alhusseini, N., et al. (2024). “Efficacy of selenium on patients undergoing cardiac surgery: A meta-analysis.” *Journal of Cardiothoracic Surgery*, 19, Article 264.

Rayman, M. P. (2012). “Selenium and human health.” *The Lancet*, 379(9822), 1256-1268.

Linder, M. C., & Hazegh-Azam, M. (1996). “Copper biochemistry and molecular biology.” *American Journal of Clinical Nutrition*, 63(5), 797S-811S.

Percival, S. S. (1998). “Copper and immunity.” *The American Journal of Clinical Nutrition*, 67(5), 1064S-1068S.

Borkow, G. (2012). “Copper as a biocidal tool.” *Current Medicinal Chemistry*, 19(5), 620-627.

Wright, J. A., et al. (2014). “The role of iron in wound healing.” *Journal of Nutrition*, 144(6), 830-836.

Coger, V., et al. (2019). “Iron in tissue repair and healing.” *Frontiers in Pharmacology*, 10, 1-8.

Iuliano, S., et al. (2021). "Calcium and protein supplementation in older adults." *BMJ*, 375, n2364.

Fischer, V., et al. (2018). "Calcium and vitamin D in bone healing." *European Cells and Materials*, 35, 265-278.

Bolland, M. J., et al. (2015). "Calcium intake and fracture risk." *BMJ*, 351, h4580.

Razzaghi, R., et al. (2017). "Effects of magnesium supplementation on wound healing." *Biological Trace Element Research*, 178(2), 301-308.

Kurmis, R., et al. (2021). "The importance of magnesium in wound management." *Wound Practice and Research*, 29(1), 4-10.

Coger, V., et al. (2019). "Magnesium levels in wound healing." *Biological Trace Element Research*, 187(2), 357-365.

Chapters 6, 7, and 8

Wischmeyer, P. E. (2018). Critical Care Clinics, 34(1), 107-125.

Carr, A. C., & Maggini, S. (2017). Nutrients, 9(11), 1211.

Holick, M. F. (2017). *The Journal of Clinical Endocrinology & Metabolism*, 102(7), 2274-2282.

Santa Mina, D., et al. (2014). BMJ Open, 4(12), e005022.

Douketis, J. D., et al. (2012). Chest, 141(2), e326S-e350S.

Practice Guidelines for Preoperative Fasting (2017). Anesthesiology, 126(3), 376-393.

Nygren, J. (2006). Current Opinion in Anaesthesiology, 19(2), 195-199.

Ljungqvist, O. (2009). Best Practice & Research Clinical Anaesthesiology, 23(4), 401-409.

Warren, J., et al. (2011). The Cochrane Database of Systematic Reviews, (2), CD004080.

Castelino, T., et al. (2016). Diseases of the Colon & Rectum, 59(12), 1164-1173.

Wischmeyer, P. E., et al. (2018). Anesthesia & Analgesia, 126(6), 1883-1895.

Gillis, C., et al. (2019) Association of Anesthetists. "Pre-operative nutrition and the elective surgical patient: why, how and what?" https://associationofanaesthetists-publications.onlinelibrary.wiley.com/doi/10.1111/anae.14506.

Hirsch, Katie R., et al. (2021). National Library of Medicine. "Pre- and Post-Surgical Nutrition for Preservation of Muscle Mass, Strength, and Functionality Following Orthopedic Surgery." https://www.ncbi.nlm.nih.gov/pmc/articles/PMC8156786/.

Chapter 9

Anderson, J. W., et al. (2009). Health benefits of dietary fiber. *Nutrition Reviews*, 67(4), 188-205. https://doi.org/10.1111/j.1753-4887.2009.00189.x

Stacewicz-Sapuntzakis, M. (2013). Dried plums and their products: Composition and health effects—An updated review. *Critical Reviews in Food Science and Nutrition*, 53(12), 1277-1302. https://doi.org/10.1080/10408398.2011.563880

Rippe, J. M., & Angelopoulos, T. J. (2012). Hydration, fluid intake, and health. *Nutrition Reviews*, 70(2), S1-S3. https://doi.org/10.1111/j.1753-4887.2012.00465.x

Röjdmark, S., et al. (1999). Influence of cytokines on appetite suppression. *Journal of Clinical Endocrinology and Metabolism*, 84(2), 465-469. https://doi.org/10.1210/jcem.84.2.5545

Michaels, A. Y., et al. (2016). Postoperative nutrition strategies. *Clinical Nutrition*, 35(3), 529-537. https://doi.org/10.1016/j.clnu.2016.03.008

Kennedy, D. O. (2016). B vitamins and the brain: Mechanisms, dose, and efficacy—A review. *Nutrients*, 8(2), 68. https://doi.org/10.3390/nu8020068

Carr, A. C., & Maggini, S. (2017). Vitamin C and immune function. *Nutrients*, 9(11), 1211. https://doi.org/10.3390/nu9111211

Arreola, R., et al. (2015). Immunomodulation and anti-inflammatory effects of garlic compounds. *Journal of Immunology Research*, 2015. https://doi.org/10.1155/2015/401630

Chapter 11

Breakfast

Amatte, Andrea. Healthy Muffins. Curated for *Heal*, 2024.

Amatte, Andrea. Savory Carrot Pudding. Curated for *Heal*, 2024.

Vera, Natasha. Apple Pie Oatmeal. Curated for *Heal*, 2024.

Vera, Natasha. Choco Chia Overnight Pudding. Curated for *Heal*, 2024.

Mandelbaum, Elizabeth Leigh. Almond Date Bars. @elizabethleigh.m, curated for *Heal*, 2024.

Mandelbaum, Elizabeth Leigh. Homemade Pumpkin Granola. @elizabethleigh.m, curated for *Heal*, 2024.

Lunch & Dinner

Vera, Natasha. Nourishing Chicken and Kale Soup. Curated for *Heal*, 2024.

Muhlstein, Ilana. Perla's Perfect Salmon; Spaghetti Squash Cacio E Pepe; Mushroom Cap Pizzas; Meatballs and Dairy-Free Cauli Mash. *Love the Food That Loves You Back* (Mango Publishing, 2020).

Vera, Natasha. Kale Pesto Pasta; Mediterranean Style Fish; Kale Quinoa Fall Bowl; Turmeric Butternut Squash Soup. Curated for *Heal*, 2024.

Klein, Dini. Enchilada Quinoa Bake; Salmon with Tahini Yogurt Sauce. Prep + Rally, 2024. www.prepandrally.com

Mandelbaum, Elizabeth Leigh. Seared Salmon Over Sauteed Garlic Spinach Tomato; Greens Soup. @elizabethleigh.m, curated for *Heal*, 2024.

Salads

Vera, Natasha. Colorful Greek Salad; Healthy Tuna Salad. Curated for *Heal*, 2024.

Muhlstein, Ilana. Fruit and Goat Cheese Salad with a Tangy Vinaigrette. *Love the Food That Loves You Back* (Mango Publishing, 2020).

Klein, Dini. Grilled Citrus Chicken Salad with Tarragon Vinaigrette. Prep + Rally, 2024. www.prepandrally.com

Healthy Desserts

Vera, Natasha. Peanut Butter & Chocolate Rice Cakes; Strawberry Yogurt Bites; Sweet Potato Brownies. Curated for *Heal*, 2024.

Amatte, Andrea. Strawberry Cheesecake. Curated for Heal, 2024.

Muhlstein, Ilana. Snickers Frowhoa; Mimi's Easy Yummy Pie. *Love the Food That Loves You Back* (Mango Publishing, 2020).

Health Tonics

Vera, Natasha. Drink the Rainbow Smoothie. Curated for *Heal*, 2024.

ACKNOWLEDGMENTS

This book, like healing itself, was not a solitary journey but rather the result of many hands, minds, and hearts working together. I am profoundly grateful to all who contributed to bringing this vision to reality.

My deepest appreciation goes to Natasha Vera, my tireless editor, whose meticulous attention to detail and unwavering dedication through countless rounds of edits shaped these pages into their final form. Alongside her, Morgane Leoni, our brilliant graphic designer, brought a visual dimension to these concepts, making complex nutritional information accessible and the recipes irresistibly appealing.

I am particularly grateful to Julie Kramer for her valuable assistance with research for this book. Her diligence and insights helped strengthen the scientific foundation of this work.

A big thank you also goes to the creators who generously contributed recipes to this book. To start off, Andrea Amatte, who is a popular recipe creator with millions of followers across the globe, thank you! Eight of her food creations are featured in the recipe section of this book. For those who want to make food that actually tastes great while still remaining healthy, you can find more of her work at @andrearecetas on Instagram.

Many delicious recipes were also provided courtesy of Ilana Muhlstein, author of Love the Food That Loves You Back (Mango Publishing), which is a fantastic clean eating cookbook you should check out next. Ilana is a Registered Dietitian Nutritionist and offers amazing meal inspiration and nutrition guidance. You can find out more about her work by booking a private session with her, purchasing her cookbook, and following her on social media at @ilanamuhlsteinrd.

Next, a heartfelt thanks to Elizabeth Leigh Mandelbaum, who is a holistic chef and a foodie content creator who has a focus on clean and simple ingredients. Her work is excellent for a whole-food focused diet like we have been talking about throughout the book. I highly recommend discovering more of her healthy creations at @elizabethleigh.m on Instagram and checking out her cookbook *Plated*.

Last, but certainly not least, thank you so much to Dini Klein. Dini is the creator of Prep + Rally (prepandrally.com) where she shares kid-friendly clean meals. Dini is a food host, former private chef, wife, and loving parent, so she knows what it is like to be busy with very little time to cook. However, she also knows how important it is to eat nutritious and wholesome meals. You can find more satisfying meal inspiration by following Dini at @ prepandrally on all socials.

To my patients, whose healing journeys inspired much of this work—thank you for trusting me with your care and for showing me, time and again, the remarkable resilience of the human body when properly nourished.

I am indebted to my office staff who assisted with the initial research phases of this project, often going above and beyond their regular duties to help compile the scientific foundation upon which this book stands.

A special thank you to my associate, Dr. Justin Karlin, for the endless discussions about nutrition and healing during our shared lunches and hikes. Your insights and questions pushed me to dig deeper and articulate these concepts more clearly.

To my mentors at the University of Miami—Dr. David Tse, Dr. Thomas Johnson, and Dr. Wendi Lee—your teachings established the foundation of my surgical career and, by extension, this book. The rigorous scientific thinking you instilled in me guided my approach to nutritional healing.

I am fortunate to have a circle of brilliant colleagues and friends who continually challenge my thinking: Dr. Ori Dastmalchi, Dr. Houman Solomon,

Dr. Sher Rabizadeh, Dr. Payam Sanjideh, Dr. Samuel Kashani, Dr. Ben Talie, Dr. Ritu Chopra, Dr. Marc Mani, Dr. Guy Massry, Dr. Babak Azizzadeh, Dr. Ramin Tabibiazar, Dr. Faryan Jalalabadi, Dr. Erez Dyan and Dr. Sirak Darbinian. Your questions, skepticism, and encouragement have strengthened both my practice and this book immeasurably.

To the countless academic researchers dedicated to nutrition science whose work I've cited throughout these pages—though we may never meet, your contributions to our understanding of how food impacts healing have made this book possible.

My heartfelt thanks go to my family, who patiently endured countless hours of my enthusiastic discussions about food and nutrition, often becoming willing (or occasionally less willing) test subjects for recipes and concepts shared in these pages. Your love and support sustain me through all my endeavors.

And to Rumi, my dog, who spent countless hours by my side as I wrote, offering silent encouragement through long writing sessions and reminding me of the importance of breaks and walks. Your presence made the solitary work of writing infinitely more joyful.

The journey to create this book has reinforced for me the very premise at its heart: healing is a collaborative process, drawing strength from many sources. My gratitude to all who have been part of this process is as boundless as the body's capacity to heal when properly nourished.

ABOUT THE AUTHOR

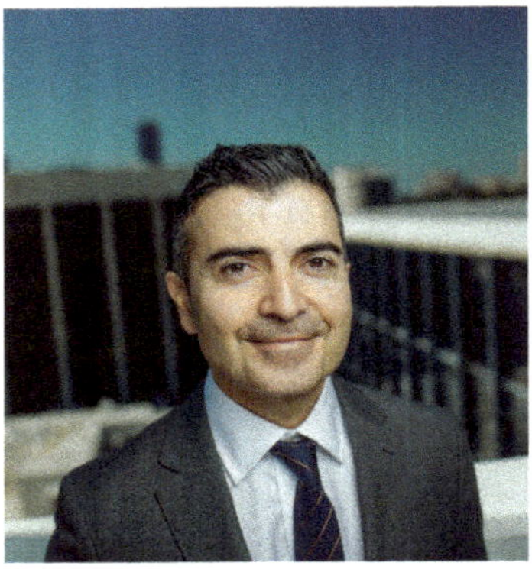

Dr. Kami Parsa is an Oculoplastic & Reconstructive Surgeon with over 20 years of specialized experience. His journey to writing this book began not in the operating room, but during a personal health crisis that transformed his understanding of the healing process.

As detailed in these pages, Dr. Parsa's perspective on recovery was profoundly altered when he discovered he had a genetic heart condition requiring open heart surgery—a diagnosis that came just as he was completing this manuscript. Having already researched nutrition for healing based on scientific evidence and his own previous experience with a hand injury, Dr. Parsa applied these principles to his own recovery. The exceptional results—being discharged just four days after major cardiac surgery—cemented his conviction in the power of nutritional healing.

A native of California, Dr. Parsa graduated with honors from the University of Southern California School of Medicine and completed his residency at USC's Doheny Eye Institute. He then pursued a two-year sub-specialty fellowship in Oculoplastic & Reconstructive Surgery at the University of Miami's Bascom Palmer Eye Institute, ranked as the nation's top program in the field.

As a Clinical Professor at USC's Department of Ophthalmology and Department of Plastic Surgery, Dr. Parsa has dedicated himself to advancing medical knowledge through research, publication, and teaching. Beyond his clinical work, he is one of the founders of Surgical Friends Foundation, a non-profit organization providing reconstructive surgery to patients without access to quality medical care.

What makes this book uniquely valuable is the rare combination of perspectives Dr. Parsa brings: the scientific rigor of a surgically trained physician, the compassionate understanding of a healthcare provider who has guided thousands through recovery, and the personal insight of someone who has applied these nutritional principles to his own healing journey with remarkable success.

When not in the operating room or writing about nutrition, Dr. Parsa enjoys globetrotting, hiking, and spending quality time with his family.

RECIPES INDEX

Breakfast

Lunch & Dinner

Salads

Sides

Healthy Desserts

Healthy Tonics

www.ingramcontent.com/pod-product-compliance
Lightning Source LLC
LaVergne TN
LVHW052113210926
848482LV00025B/554
* 9 7 9 8 9 9 3 2 4 1 2 0 3 *